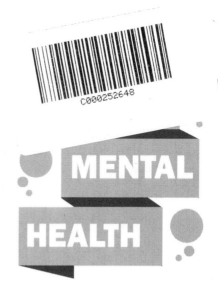

MENTAL HEALTH

MEETING THE MENTAL HEALTH NEEDS

OF YOUNG CHILDREN 0–5 YEARS

POSITIVE MENTAL HEALTH

This new series of texts presents a modern and comprehensive set of evidence-based strategies for promoting positive mental health in educational settings. There is a growing prevalence of mental ill-health among children and young people within a context of funding cuts, strained services and a lack of formal training for practitioners. The series recognises the complexity of the issues involved, the vital role that educational professionals play, and the current education and health policy frameworks, in order to provide practical guidance backed up by the latest research.

Our titles are also available in a range of electronic formats. To order, or for details of our bulk discounts, please go to our website www. criticalpublishing.com or contact our distributor, NBN International, 10 Thornbury Road, Plymouth PL6 7PP, telephone 01752 202301 or email orders@nbninternational.com.

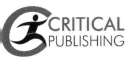

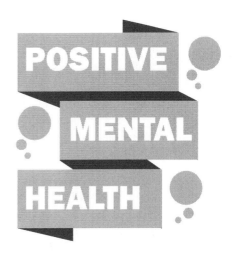

MEETING THE MENTAL HEALTH NEEDS

OF YOUNG CHILDREN 0–5 YEARS

Jonathan Glazzard, Marie Potter and Samuel Stones

First published in 2019 by Critical Publishing Ltd

British Library Cataloguing in Publication Data
A CIP record for this book is available from the British Library

ISBN: 978-1-912508-89-1

This book is also available in the following e-book formats:
MOBI ISBN: 978-1-912508-90-7
EPUB ISBN: 978-1-912508-91-4
Adobe e-book ISBN: 978-1-912508-92-1

Cover and text design by Out of House Limited
Project Management by Newgen Publishing UK
Printed and bound in Great Britain by 4edge, Essex

Critical Publishing
3 Connaught Road
St Albans
AL3 5RX

www.criticalpublishing.com

Paper from responsible sources

✚ CONTENTS

MEET THE SERIES EDITOR AND AUTHORS PAGE VII

INTRODUCTION PAGE 1

+MEET THE SERIES EDITOR AND AUTHORS

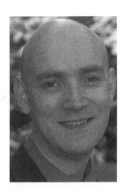

JONATHAN GLAZZARD

Jonathan Glazzard is series editor for *Positive Mental Health.* He is Professor of Teacher Education at Leeds Beckett University and is the professor attached to the Carnegie Centre of Excellence for Mental Health in Schools. He teaches across a range of QTS and non-QTS programmes and is an experienced teacher educator.

MARIE POTTER

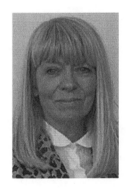

Marie Potter is a Senior Lecturer in the Institute of Childhood and Education at Leeds Trinity University. She is the Programme Leader for the BA (Hons) Early Childhood Studies and BA (Hons) Education Studies and a dissertation supervisor on the MA in Education. Marie is an experienced HE lecturer with a background in early years, she previously worked as the manager of an early years setting and as a freelance consultant specialising in emotional development, play and learning and behaviour management; she also worked as an early years adviser and CPD trainer for Leeds Education Authority and Social Services.

SAMUEL STONES

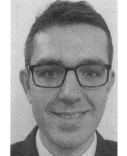

Samuel Stones is associate leader of maths, computing, economics and business at a secondary academy in North Yorkshire. He works with initial teacher training students in university and school contexts and is an experienced educator and examiner. He supports a teacher well-being and mental health working group.

✚ INTRODUCTION

The Early Years Foundation Stage provides a unique opportunity to support children's holistic development. The prime areas of learning underpin the specific areas and are therefore critical to children's learning. Children cannot thrive if they have poor well-being, low self-worth and are unable to regulate their behaviour and emotions. Effective practitioners know that all children are unique. They learn at different rates, have different strengths and interests and therefore require varying levels of support. Some children will have endured adverse childhood experiences, including abuse, neglect and parental conflict and separation. These experiences can have a long-lasting detrimental impact on their mental health and on their learning and development. Effective early years practitioners understand the importance of establishing positive, warm and trusting relationships with children. They recognise the need for children to experience a sense of belonging in the setting and they understand the importance of giving children agency. High-quality early years settings can reduce the effects of adverse childhood experiences but cannot necessarily eradicate the impact that these experiences have had on children's development.

This book provides an overview of the risk and protective factors that result in mental ill-health in the early years. The themes of attachment, resilience and self-regulation are explored from a theoretical perspective and in relation to the practical implications for early years practitioners. Case studies are used to exemplify some of the issues and to illuminate effective practice.

Children's experiences of transition can affect their mental health. Transitioning from the home environment to the pre-school setting can be traumatic for some children. Skilled practitioners will be aware that while some children are more resilient than others and are able to adapt to change more quickly, some children take longer to adapt and require more support during times of transition. Demonstrating kindness, empathy and treating children with respect are simple ways of supporting children through difficult transitions.

This book recognises the critical role of learning through play in the early years. It emphasises the value of adult intervention in children's play to extend learning and development and the role of play in supporting all

1

aspects of children's development. Providing children with rich, stimulating learning opportunities through play can support the development of self-regulation skills, which are vital for positive mental health. At the same time, the book acknowledges that the value of play-based pedagogy in the Reception year has been questioned by Ofsted. In Chapter 7, it is argued that a focus on 'schoolification' in the early years is a misinformed move, which could have significant and detrimental effects on young children's mental health.

Children in the early years can experience a range of forms of mental ill-health. This book addresses the main mental health needs and provides an overview of the signs and symptoms of mental ill-health. It is argued that the development of a social and emotional curriculum, which provides children with the skills that they need to develop positive social interactions, empathy, resilience and emotional regulation, is an essential aspect of the early years curriculum, which can support positive well-being in the early years.

We hope you enjoy reading this book.

Jonathan Glazzard, Marie Potter and Samuel Stones

✚ CHAPTER 1

FACTORS THAT PUT CHILDREN AT RISK

PROFESSIONAL LINKS

This chapter addresses the following:

Department for Education (2017) *Statutory Framework for the Early Years Foundation Stage: Setting the Standards for Learning, Development and Care for Children from Birth to Five*. London: DfE.

CHAPTER OBJECTIVES

By the end of this chapter you will understand:

+ the risk factors that can result in children developing mental ill-health;

+ your role as a practitioner in mitigating these risk factors.

INTRODUCTION

This chapter addresses the risk factors that increase the likelihood that children will develop mental ill-health. Some of these factors are related to adverse childhood experiences that children are exposed to in the home and the community. While you cannot always eradicate these from children's lives, there are things that you can do within the context of the early years setting to compensate for the effects of these adverse experiences. This chapter addresses the individual, family and community factors that increase the risk of childhood mental ill-health. It also addresses the role of practitioners within the setting in mitigating some of these risks.

INDIVIDUAL FACTORS

GENETIC INFLUENCES

As a practitioner, you must understand the ways in which genes influence children's learning. Developing this understanding allows the children you teach to thrive, become more fulfilled and thus experience positive mental health. Furthermore, children are individuals with their own traits, temperament, needs and preferences (Asbury and Plomin, 2013). Therefore, we need to acknowledge that more of the same is unlikely to be the most suitable approach for most children.

If a child is not learning in the same way as other children or is not making the progress they are expected to, you must adapt your approach and use your knowledge of children as individuals. This is likely to involve making decisions to allocate or target resources and support at specific children while withdrawing these from others. Through understanding the needs of all children, education can support all children and ensure that genetic influences are not a negative barrier to a child achieving successful outcomes (Asbury and Plomin, 2013).

Children may also seek learning opportunities on the basis of their preferences, which have been shaped by their genes (Asbury and Plomin, 2013), and as a practitioner you must look for and respond to these calls to maximise children's chances of fulfilling their potential across all area of learning and development in the Early Years Foundation Stage framework. Doing so personalises a child's learning, provides an inclusive environment for all and allows positive mental health to permeate the early years.

While research studies have confirmed that genetic factors have a substantial influence on children's learning (Schumacher et al, 2007), the debate of nature and nurture remains critical. This debate continues to produce evidence that demonstrates the impact of environmental loci (Hart et al, 2014). These include the children themselves, as well as practitioners and parents who can work together and overcome many of the challenges of genetic influence (Hart et al, 2013).

LEARNING DISABILITIES

Children with learning disabilities have a higher risk of developing mental ill-health compared to the general population (Hackett et al, 2011). It has been argued that they are six times more likely to develop mental health difficulties (Emerson and Hatton, 2007), and for those with learning disabilities who are placed in the care system the likelihood of developing mental ill-health may be even higher than this (Taggart et al, 2007).

Children with learning disabilities may experience multiple forms of disadvantage. They are more likely to experience social deprivation and adverse childhood experiences. They may also have multiple and complex disabilities, and this can affect their feelings of self-worth. The rates of anxiety disorders in children with autistic spectrum conditions range from 11 per cent to 84 per cent (Brookman-Frazee et al, 2018) and research suggests that children with autism often access mental health services due to demonstrating challenging behaviour (Brookman-Frazee et al, 2012).

FOETAL ALCOHOL SPECTRUM DISORDER

Foetal alcohol spectrum disorder (FASD) is a term used to describe the range of mental and physical birth defects caused by alcohol exposure during pregnancy. Alcohol disrupts foetal development and FASD refers

5

to the permanent brain damage that results from this pre-birth exposure (Catterick and Curran, 2014). The deficits caused by FASD are not fully understood, although exploring and understanding these is critical in supporting those affected (Rasmussen, 2005). Children with foetal alcohol spectrum disorder may exhibit physical anomalies including vision, hearing and motor problems (Stratton et al, 1996).

As a practitioner, there any many strategies that you can use to support children with FASD and in doing so ensure their inclusion and thus support their positive mental health. Using children's names to make sure that you have their attention before you speak to them can support those experiencing hearing difficulties. You should also use concisely chunked instructions and simple language to support children with cognitive and motor difficulties. Where possible, practitioners should also share with parents and carers any common language that can be used both at the child's home and during their interactions at school.

Practitioners must also acknowledge the strengths and interests of those with FASD when considering their own planning, as this supports the provision of an inclusive environment for children who may otherwise by overwhelmed by sensory stimulation. Likewise, multisensory experiences can be based around students' sensory strengths and these can promote positive mental health (Blackburn, 2010).

RESILIENCE

Children who are resilient can 'bounce-back' from adversity. Their response to a negative experience is to acknowledge it, recover from it and then learn from it. Resilient children are not permanently negatively affected by adverse experiences. They can move forward from situations and experiences to lead positive and fulfilling lives. Children who are less resilient may be negatively affected by adverse experiences for longer. It may take longer for them to recover from adversity and they may be permanently negatively affected by it. A variety of terms are used synonymously to denote resilience. These include *perseverance*, *grit*, *determination*, *stickability*, *bounce-back* and *character*.

Resilience in children is affected by their sense of self-worth. Those with a high self-worth may be able to recover from negative experiences more quickly than those with low self-worth. Confidence is also important. Children who lack confidence may take longer to recover from adversity compared to those who demonstrate high confidence. Additionally, children who adapt well to changes in their lives may be more resilient when they experience adversity compared to those who find change difficult.

CRITICAL QUESTIONS

+ How can practitioners promote resilience in the early years?

+ In what ways can practitioners support the development of physical and social and emotional resilience?

+ How can practitioners promote resilience in relation to perseverance after defeat; for example, when completing tasks such as building towers with bricks or completing jigsaws?

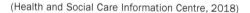

In 2017, 6.8 per cent of boys aged 2–4 years had mental ill-health.

In 2017, 4.2 per cent of girls aged 2–4 years had mental ill-health.

(Health and Social Care Information Centre, 2018)

CRITICAL QUESTIONS

+ Why do you think that mental ill-health is more common in boys than girls?

+ What are the implications of this for early years settings?

FAMILY AND COMMUNITY FACTORS

Risk factors that detrimentally impact on young children's mental health include:

+ parental conflict;

+ family breakdown;

+ hostile or rejecting relationships;

+ abuse and neglect;

+ parental psychiatric distress;

+ parental criminality;

+ parental alcoholism;

+ death and loss;

+ children moving into care, being fostered or adopted;

+ poverty or socio-economic disadvantage.

As a practitioner you will need to be aware of which children are exposed to these risk factors. You will need to be aware of changes of mood and behaviour that may indicate that there are problems at home. Very young children may not be able to communicate their distress verbally. This is where key workers are important, as they will be attuned to the child's usual behaviour and in a position to know when that changes. Sometimes children may alert you to situations at home, although this is rare. If you suspect that a child is being abused or neglected, you should always follow the guidance in the setting's safeguarding policy. It is never acceptable to do nothing.

It is important that you provide a safe, nurturing environment for all children, but particularly for children who are experiencing adverse circumstances at home. The circumstances at home may result in the child developing low self-worth, high levels of anxiety or stress, depression, reduced confidence and social isolation. Adverse circumstances at home can also result in children developing social, emotional and behavioural difficulties.

Some children who experience adverse circumstances might be capable of working at or above age-related expectations across all areas of learning and development. It is important to have high expectations of all children in your care. If their progress suddenly stalls or declines, this might be an indication that the child is experiencing mental ill-health as a result of adverse experiences. You will need to observe the child in a range of contexts to ascertain whether there is sufficient evidence of mental ill-health or whether their mood and/or behaviour is triggered by something specific in the setting.

It is important that you do not stereotype families. Although adverse childhood circumstances take place in families that experience social deprivation, remember that abuse, neglect, domestic violence, family breakdown and parental criminality cut across all social backgrounds. Forms of neglect, for example, may vary across different social backgrounds but the impact on the child is still negative. Children may appear to be well-fed, clean and looked after, but sometimes these factors can mask adverse experiences that detrimentally impact on children.

Community factors also increase the likelihood of children developing mental ill-health. Socio-economic disadvantage has been associated with exposure to adverse childhood experiences that can increase the risk of childhood mental illness. In addition, community-related factors such as homelessness, national or community conflict can also increase the risk of children developing mental ill-health.

According to the Mental Health Foundation (2016, p 57):

A growing body of evidence, mainly from high-income countries, has shown that there is a strong socioeconomic gradient in mental health, with people of lower socioeconomic status having a higher likelihood of developing and experiencing mental health problems. In other words, social inequalities in society are strongly linked to mental health inequalities.

Thus, socio-economic disadvantage acts as a psychosocial stressor and can have a detrimental impact on children's mental health and well-being. It is also associated with worse parental mental health, which is, in turn, a strong risk factor for poor child mental health and well-being (Education Policy Institute, 2018). Additionally, adverse childhood experiences, including experiences of abuse, neglect and parental conflict have a known and significant detrimental effect on children and young people's mental health. These include trauma, poor attachment, parental alcohol and drug abuse, domestic violence, neglect and abuse (House of Commons, 2018).

CASE STUDY

Luke was four years old. He was attending the school nursery attached to the local community primary school and his father was an alcoholic. Consequently, Luke was, in the main, cared for by his mother. His parents argued on a daily basis and arguments frequently carried on into the night. Sometimes the arguments became physical. Often, Luke's sleep was broken, and he was tired in the mornings, frequently resulting in him not wanting to attend the nursery. Luke was worried about his parents and he was reluctant to leave them during the day. He started to demonstrate uncooperative behaviour in the nursery and he became physically aggressive with practitioners and other children. Often, Luke would socially isolate himself away from other children and he pushed them away when his space was invaded. His progress across all areas of learning and development was below age-related expectations and his key worker, Emily, was concerned about his well-being.

Emily focused on establishing warm, positive and trusting relationships with Luke. She demonstrated unconditional positive regard towards him and she praised him when she noticed something positive. Sanctions were not applied, even when Luke demonstrated physical aggression. Emily decided to develop a social and emotional intervention programme for Luke and a small number of children in the nursery who were working below age-related expectations in personal, social and emotional development. The intervention focused on feelings. The children were taught, over several weeks, to name feelings and they were introduced to some strategies to regulate their own feelings. Emily also focused on developing their understanding of how other children's feelings can be affected by things that are done to them or said to them. Sessions were interactive; Emily used a range of stories that focused on feelings and puppets. There was a strong focus on empathy, including how to show kindness to others. Emily then designed a series of sessions to focus on developing social skills. These sessions included themes such as turn-taking, sharing and being a good communicator.

After a term, all the children who had participated in the intervention, including Luke, were working at age-related expectations in personal, social and emotional development.

FACTORS RELATED TO THE SETTING

Establishing warm, positive and trusting relationships with all children is critical to develop children's self-worth and confidence. Negative or hostile relationships can increase the likelihood of children becoming stressed, anxious or depressed and social learning theory suggests that children can imitate the behaviours that they observe.

Children who feel included in the setting and who experience a sense of belonging are less likely to develop mental ill-health. Displays and resources that reflect the lives and identities of children will facilitate a sense of inclusion. Young children often arrive in settings without the social, emotional, language and communication skills that they need to enable them to thrive within the setting. Responding to their behaviour through establishing sanctions is not an effective way of helping young children to learn how to adjust their behaviour to the context of the setting. Your role as a practitioner is to recognise that children have often not developed the social and emotional skills they need but with the right support they can learn to adjust their behaviour.

Effective settings in the early years provide opportunities for both adult-directed and child-initiated learning. Learning through play is more effective when practitioners intervene in children's play to further develop their knowledge and skills. Children need exposure to child-initiated, adult-supported and adult-directed play as well as adult-directed learning. Achieving a balance between adult-directed and independent learning is crucial to support children's learning and development. Providing children with access to a language and literacy rich environment in the early years will also facilitate the development of reading and writing skills. Children should have frequent opportunities to listen to stories and poems and to handle books. Providing children with choice in their activities will reduce stress and anxiety, although providing them with too much choice can restrict learning and development. Children need to be exposed to unfamiliar challenges to develop the skill of resilience. Practitioners can initially scaffold their learning in these tasks to support children to develop their skills and confidence.

CRITICAL QUESTIONS

+ Should the pedagogical approaches adopted in the early years be adapted for children in the Reception year? Explain your answer.

+ Do you agree that formal learning in the early years can result in children developing mental ill-health? Explain your answer.

+ How can resilience be developed in the early years?

CASE STUDY

Jane was a practitioner working in the early years in an area of social deprivation. She had identified a group of children at the start of the academic year who were displaying signs of conduct disorder. They were defiant to the practitioners in the setting and destructive to the physical environment. Other children in the setting had started to replicate the negative behaviours that they had observed. Jane noticed that the children were not using the resources in the continuous provision appropriately. Resources were not handled with care, were frequently broken and the children did not persist with self-chosen activities.

Jane realised that the children's progress across all areas of learning and development in the Early Years Foundation Stage framework would be detrimentally affected by the children's skills in personal, social and emotional development. The children did not know how to play, and they were not able to follow the rules of the setting. Children frequently moved from one activity to another without engaging in any meaningful learning opportunities and this meant that they were not exploiting the learning opportunities that were available to them.

Jane decided that all practitioners in the setting would be responsible for locating themselves in specific areas of continuous provision. The role of the practitioners was to model how to use the resources in the provision, how to play and persist with self-chosen activities. The practitioners also modelled vocabulary, language and communication skills while playing alongside the children. This adult intervention in children's play was a way of scaffolding the children's learning. Initially, the children were restricted to using two areas of provision; for example, they were permitted to move between the sand area and the water area. Using a planning board, they had access to different areas of provision on different days, but on a single day they were required to learn in two areas.

Over a period of four weeks the children demonstrated improvements in their behaviour. They had started to use the resources appropriately and they were persisting for longer in self-chosen activities. Eventually, Jane extended the range of areas to three and then to four. After seven weeks, Jane was confident that the children could have free access to all areas of provision and adult intervention in child-initiated play was reduced. Their behaviour improved, and they demonstrated progress in all areas of learning and development.

Research demonstrates that the physical, social and emotional environment in the setting impacts on children's physical, emotional and mental health and well-being as well as impacting on their learning and development (Jamal et al, 2013).

In addition, research suggests that relationships between staff and children, and between children, are critical in promoting well-being and in helping to engender a sense of belonging to the setting (Calear and Christensen, 2010).

● In 2017, 3.1 per cent of boys aged 2–4 years had a conduct disorder.

● In 2017, 1.9 per cent of girls aged 2–4 years had a conduct disorder.

(Health and Social Care Information Centre, 2018)

CRITICAL QUESTIONS

+ Why do you think conduct disorders are more prevalent in boys than girls?

+ What are the implications of this for early years settings?

SUMMARY

This chapter has identified the risk factors that increase the likelihood of children developing mental ill-health. The role and influence of foetal alcohol disorder syndrome, genetics and learning disabilities has been explored and the impact of these on children's mental health has been highlighted. Practical strategies have been provided to equip practitioners with a toolkit to compensate for the effects of children's adverse experiences. Individual, family and community factors that increase the risk of childhood mental ill-health have also been explained.

CHECKLIST

This chapter has addressed:

✓ the risk factors that increase the likelihood of children developing mental ill-health;

✓ the importance of practitioners responding to the needs of children affected by foetal alcohol disorder syndrome, genetic influences and learning disabilities;

✓ the strategies available to you as a practitioner in supporting students with diverse needs;

✓ the individual and family and community factors that increase the likelihood of children developing mental ill-health.

FURTHER READING

Asbury, K and Plomin, R (2013) *G is for Genes: The Impact of Genetics on Education and Achievement (Understanding Children's Worlds)*. Oxford: Wiley Blackwell.

Catterick, M and Curran, L (2014) *Understanding Fetal Alcohol Spectrum Disorder: A Guide to FASD for Parents, Carers and Professionals*. London: Jessica Kingsley Publishers.

✚ CHAPTER 2

THE SIGNIFICANCE OF ATTACHMENT IN THE EARLY YEARS

PROFESSIONAL LINKS

This chapter addresses the following:

The Early Years Foundation Stage framework states that *'each child must be assigned a key person. Their role is to help ensure that every child's care is tailored to meet their individual needs to help the child become familiar with the setting, offer a settled relationship for the child and build a relationship with their parents'* (DfE, 2017, para 3.27).

CHAPTER OBJECTIVES

By the end of this chapter you will understand:

+ the assumptions underpinning attachment theory;

+ the implications of attachment theory for practitioners who work in early years.

INTRODUCTION

This chapter addresses the role of attachment in supporting children's well-being. The relationship that a child establishes with their primary carer is critical to their subsequent development. If the relationship is strong and loving, children are able to flourish. If the relationship is hostile or broken, this can have a significant long-term effect on the child's social and emotional development. The quality of the relationship between the child and their primary carer is influenced by the quality of the interactions between both and the extent to which the carer addresses the child's needs. If a child's physiological, safety and emotional needs are not met, this can result in the child feeling unloved. If the child receives negative feedback from their primary carer, this can lead to feelings of low self-worth. If the child is separated from their primary carer, they can experience a sense of rejection, which impacts on self-worth and confidence.

The quality of the attachment between the child and their primary carer is not related to the child's social background. Children from deprived social backgrounds can still experience positive attachments if they are loved, nurtured and provided with positive feedback. In addition, children from more affluent backgrounds can experience disrupted attachments if they do not spend sufficient time with their primary carer.

WHAT IS ATTACHMENT?

Attachment refers to the bond that a child establishes with their primary carer, usually the mother. Attachment theory emerged from Bowlby's clinical observations in his seminal study of 44 'delinquent' children. Based on these observations, Bowlby concluded that a broken mother–child relationship in the first three years of life leads to children becoming emotionally withdrawn (Bowlby, 1940). Bowlby emphasised the impact of physical separation from the primary carer and concluded that the physical disruption of the bond between the child and the carer may have a detrimental effect on subsequent personality development. According to Bowlby, even minor separation experiences could have a detrimental effect on the healthy development of young children (Bowlby, 1960).

Bowlby argued that the emotional bond between child and mother was the basis for all further social development (Bowlby, 1939). He stated that:

the evidence is now such that it leaves no room for doubt regarding the general propositions – that the prolonged deprivation of the young child of maternal care may have grave and far-reaching effects on his character and so on the whole of his future life.

(Bowlby, 1952, p 46)

Bowlby also believed that it was essential for mental health *'that the infant and young child should experience a warm, intimate, and continuous relationship with his mother (or permanent mother-substitute)'* (Bowlby, 1952, p 11).

Your knowledge of the child's family background may give you some insight into the quality of the attachments between the child and their primary carer. Where possible, you should undertake a home visit to observe the interactions that take place between the child and the adult. For children who have developed weak attachments, or for those who have been deprived of material care through physical separation from their mother, it is particularly important that you develop positive, warm and nurturing relationships with them to provide them with the emotional security that is lacking in the home. As a key worker you may need to spend more time interacting with these children so that they can start to establish a bond with you. Children can and do form strong attachments with practitioners who form positive, caring and consistent relationships with them.

In the case of young children, transferring attachment from the main carer to the practitioner for infants and toddlers can be a more difficult event for everyone. Sometimes the assumption is made that the crying which may occur is because that's what babies do. It can be helpful for all concerned to understand that often infants cry to alert the parent and keep them close by, like lambs in the field calling for their mothers. When they are handed over to a stranger they may try to use that alert system. It might be better to have a policy to allow the main carer to initially stay and play with the child in the setting where this is possible. The next stage is to hand over the child to the key worker with the carer sitting at a distance. The carer can leave the room for a short time until eventually the handover is effective. This ensures the child is calm and feels safe, rather than feeling unhappy and insecure.

CRITICISMS OF ATTACHMENT THEORY

Attachment theory has been criticised because of Bowlby's emphasis on the mother rather than the primary caregiver. In today's modern society, children are born into diverse families, including those with same-sex parents. The emphasis on the mother as the key figure within attachment underplays the critical role that other carers can have on children's development. These include:

+ foster carers;

+ same-sex parents;

+ parents who adopt;

+ single fathers who take responsibility for parenting;

+ fathers who are the primary carer while the mother works.

CRITICAL QUESTIONS

+ What factors might result in weak attachments developing between the child and their primary carer?

+ In your setting, how do you identify children with attachment needs?

+ How do you support children with attachment needs in your setting?

55 per cent of children with oppositional defiant disorder or conduct disorder demonstrate signs of insecure attachment.

(www.nice.org.uk/guidance/ng26/documents/childrens-attachment-full-guideline2)

SIGNS OF POOR ATTACHMENTS

Attachment disorder is a term used to describe disorders of mood, behaviour and social relationships arising from weak, disrupted or non-existent attachments between the child and their primary carer. Attachment difficulties are usually always caused by inappropriate parenting and genetic studies show minimal genetic influence on attachment patterns. Attachment bonds become evident between six and nine months. If the attachment with the carer is not established during this critical period of development then this can result in the child developing attachment disorder.

Common signs of attachment disorder include:

+ aversion to physical contact or physical affection;

+ poor behaviour, such as disobedience, defiance and anger;

+ avoiding eye-contact;

+ non-verbal communication;

+ crying and not smiling;

+ interacting with strangers but not with the primary carer;

+ showing no signs of distress when they are left alone.

TYPES OF ATTACHMENT

Mary Ainsworth's work has been seminal in helping practitioners and academics to identify different attachment behaviours. The research study that resulted in these categories of attachment is stated in the research box below.

The Strange Situation Procedure is Ainsworth's best-known contribution to attachment theory (Ainsworth et al, 1978). In the experiment eight episodes were observed.

1. The child was first taken to a strange environment with its mother.

2. Next a stranger enters the room to join the mother and the child.

3. The mother then leaves the room and the child is left with the stranger.

4. The mother then returns to the room to join the child and the stranger.

5. The stranger then leaves the room and the child is left with the mother.

6. The mother also leaves the room and the child is alone in the room.

7. Then the stranger returns to the room to join the child.

8. Finally the mother returns to the room to join the child and the stranger.

The child was observed during each of these scenarios using a two-way mirror.

From this experiment three types of attachment behaviour were observed.

+ Secure attachments: when the mother leaves the room, the child becomes distressed and experiences separation anxiety. The child avoids the stranger when they are alone with them (stranger anxiety) but the child is friendly towards the stranger when the mother returns. When the mother returns to the room the child is happy.

+ Resistant attachments: the child shows signs of intense distress when the mother leaves the room and when left alone with the stranger the child shows signs of fear. When the mother returns to the room the child approaches the mother but subsequently resists contact. The child may reject the mother by pushing her away.

+ Avoidant attachments: the child shows no sign of distress when the mother leaves the room. The child is happy to interact with the stranger when left alone with them. The child shows little or no interest in the mother when the mother returns to the room.

CRITICAL QUESTIONS

+ What factors may result in the child demonstrating secure attachments with their mother?

+ Why do you think the child with resistant attachments pushes the mother away?

+ What factors might result in the child developing avoidant attachments?

+ In your setting, which children demonstrate secure, resistant or avoidant attachments?

+ What are the implications of these different types of attachments for early years practitioners?

CASE STUDY

Rameena was three years of age. Her mother was sent to prison for a six-year sentence before Rameena was born. Following her birth, she was cared for by her grandparents. Rameena visited the prison during the initial four months of her life but then her mother decided that the environment of the prison was not appropriate for her daughter. Rameena became upset when she was separated from her mother during these visits and consequently it was decided that Rameena would make no further visits to the prison.

Rameena initially attended a local playgroup before she started pre-school. Ameena was assigned as her key worker. Ameena noticed quite quickly that Rameena demonstrated signs of potential conduct disorder. She was frequently defiant and refused to comply with requests. She often walked away from Ameena and sometimes she physically pushed her away. She preferred to play alone, and she rejected child or adult interventions in her play. She frequently threw resources around the room, which she refused to pick up. She refused to sit at the snack table to eat and she had started to rip up the story books in the reading area. Rameena cried frequently and she was rarely seen smiling.

Ameena requested a meeting with Rameena's grandparents. She explained her concerns about Rameena's social and emotional development and she invited them to share their perspectives on Rameena's behaviour at home. Rameena's grandparents acknowledged that they had also experienced similar behaviour in the home and that they were struggling to manage it.

Ameena suggested that a pet might be a positive addition to the family so that Rameena could develop an attachment to it. It was agreed that a dog would be purchased and that Rameena would take some responsibility for caring for the animal. The family purchased a dog and decided to name him Sebastian. Rameena instantly loved Sebastian and she started to bring photographs of him into the setting. Ameena used this as an opportunity to establish positive relationships with Rameena. Together, they looked at the photographs and talked about Sebastian every day. Ameena was keen to find out about the dog and to use this as an opportunity to promote Rameena's learning and development.

Ameena decided to create a daily diary for Rameena to share with Sebastian each night. She took photographs of Rameena engaging in various activities during the day and placed these in the diary. Samples of Rameena's work were also placed in the diary. Rameena took the diary home every night and shared it with Sebastian. This task motivated Rameena to engage in various activities during the day but also helped to develop positive relationships between Rameena and Ameena.

Data from 2017 on children aged 2–4 indicate that:

- 1.8 per cent of children from the least deprived areas had a behavioural disorder compared to 3.3 per cent from the most deprived areas;

- 1.8 per cent had a behavioural disorder in London compared to 3.6 per cent in the north of England;

- 5.4 per cent of children with a behavioural disorder were in families in receipt of state benefits compared to 1 per cent in families in receipt of no benefits;

- 1.8 per cent of children with behavioural disorders were from high or middle income families compared to 4.5 per cent from the lowest earning families.

(Health and Social Care Information Centre, 2018)

CRITICAL QUESTIONS

+ How might you explain the differences in the statistics?

+ Are these statistics representative of children in your setting?

+ What are the implications of these statistics for your own setting?

+ Do all children with behavioural disorder also have attachment disorders? Explain your response.

THE IMPACT OF POOR ATTACHMENTS

Children's early interactions with their primary caregivers form a 'blueprint' in the child's mind for how relationships operate. If children experience rejection from their parents or hostile interactions, there is a danger that they will replicate these interactions in other relationships. Social learning theory suggests that children tend to imitate the behaviours they observe. In addition, if children have not got strong attachments with their primary caregiver, this can impact detrimentally on how they view themselves. They might demonstrate low self-worth and low confidence, and this can impact detrimentally on their development across all areas of learning. Children who have experienced rejection might find it more difficult to establish social relationships with others. In particular, they might find it difficult to trust other people. They might demonstrate conduct disorders and show signs of poor emotional regulation.

Maslow's hierarchy of needs is a useful theoretical framework to help you understand the impact of unfulfilled needs on children's development (Maslow, 1943, 1954). Maslow stated that basic physiological needs such as food, water, warmth and rest need to be met first. If children's basic needs are unmet, this can impact on the quality of the attachments that they form with their primary carer. Next, children need to feel safe. After that, they need to feel loved and experience a sense of belonging. If these needs are unmet, children may feel rejected by their primary carer and this can have a detrimental impact on the quality of the attachments. The next level of needs are 'self' needs. Children need to have a positive sense of self-worth and good self-esteem to be able to thrive and if the earlier needs are not met, then this can have a detrimental effect on the child's sense of self. Finally, all of these needs need to be met before the child can achieve their full potential. Maslow referred to this as *self-actualisation*. Children who have not established secure attachments may not have had their basic physiological and safety needs met. They may not feel loved, and hostile and rejecting interactions from the primary carer may result in feelings of low self-worth. These factors can affect children's abilities to achieve their full potential across all areas of learning and development in the Early Years Foundation Stage framework.

Attachment disorder symptoms are more common in children who have been exposed to abuse or neglect and in children who have been separated from prior caregivers. Children in foster care have a higher risk of developing attachment disorder. This is mainly due to earlier experiences of abuse or neglect in their biological families, experiences of unsatisfactory care in care homes, and/or the separation from primary caregivers.

(Minnis et al, 2006)

CASE STUDY

Sam was four years old. His mother was alcohol-dependent and his father was drug-dependent. At the age of two, social care services agreed to separate Sam from his parents and to place him into local authority foster care. Following this, his behaviour at home had started to deteriorate and Sam was frequently defiant to his foster carers. He was in the Reception year at his local school and the practitioners were struggling to manage Sam's behaviour. He refused to sit still on the carpet, he disobeyed instructions from practitioners and he had started to demonstrate signs of physical aggression towards other children. He had low self-worth and he often referred to himself as *'stupid'*. Sam found it difficult to establish positive social relationships with other children and he preferred to play alone rather than playing with his peers. His profile of achievement across all areas of the Early Years Foundation Stage framework was below the standard that was expected for his age.

The key worker decided to implement several strategies to support Sam.

+ An individual reward system was implemented to reward good behaviour.

+ A visual timetable was developed to provide Sam with clear routine.

+ A visual slider was used during structured tasks: it included the words 'start' and 'stop' at opposite ends of a line and a moveable arrow so that Sam could see how much progress he had made through a task.

+ A visual 'thermometer' was introduced to support Sam in regulating his own feelings: the bottom of the thermometer represented the feeling of 'calm' and the top of the thermometer represented the feeling of wanting to 'explode'. Other feelings were represented in between these two extremes including feelings of being 'irritated' or 'annoyed'. Sam was allowed to use the thermometer to indicate changes to his feelings at different times of the day. When his key worker noticed that his mood was changing, she used this as an opportunity to discuss his feelings and this supported Sam in regulating his feelings.

+ A 'circle of friends' approach was implemented as a strategy to improve Sam's self-worth. Sam chose three children who he felt he could be friends with. Each week they met with Sam and his key worker to identify positive traits about him.

+ The key worker identified that Sam had an interest in spiders so she creatively built spiders into as many curriculum areas as possible. Age-appropriate books were purchased on spiders for Sam to read and opportunities to investigate spiders in the outdoor area were integrated into the curriculum.

SUMMARY

This chapter has highlighted the role of attachment in supporting children's well-being. It has explored the value of a child establishing relationships with their primary carers and identifies the long-term effects of these on the child's social and emotional development. The chapter also explains the importance of interaction between a child and their primary carer. Children's physiological, safety and emotional needs are discussed and the importance of these is emphasised. The quality of the attachment between the child and their primary carer is illustrated and the chapter has emphasised that children from deprived social backgrounds can still experience positive attachments if they are loved, nurtured and provided with positive feedback.

CHECKLIST

This chapter has addressed:

✓ the impact of poor attachments on children's development;

✓ the types of attachment and the research underpinning these;

✓ the implications of attachment theory for practitioners working in the early years.

FURTHER READING

Elfer, P Goldschmied, E and Selleck, D (2012) *Key Persons in the Early Years*. Oxon: Routledge.

✚ CHAPTER 3

DEVELOPING RESILIENCE IN THE EARLY YEARS

PROFESSIONAL LINKS

This chapter addresses the following:

Department for Education (2017) *Statutory Framework for the Early Years Foundation Stage: Setting the Standards for Learning, Development and Care for Children from Birth to Five*. London: DfE.

CHAPTER OBJECTIVES

By the end of this chapter you will understand:

+ what is meant by the concept of resilience;

+ how to develop resilience in an early years setting.

INTRODUCTION

The first overarching principle of the Early Years Foundation Stage framework is that *'every child is a unique child, who is constantly learning and can be resilient, capable, confident and self-assured'* (DfE, 2017, p 6). The second principle is that children should *'learn to be strong and independent through positive relationships'* (DfE, 2017, p 6). Both of these principles reflect current discourses on childhood that position children as strong and capable social actors who are able to 'bounce-back' from adverse childhood experiences. However, perspectives on childhood have changed significantly over time and discourses on childhood have shaped perspectives on resilience. This chapter will explore some of the tensions associated with resilience and highlight strategies for developing resilience in the early years setting.

PERSPECTIVES ON CHILDHOOD AND RESILIENCE

Over 20 years ago it was argued that:

Children are arguably more hemmed in by surveillance and social regulation than ever before. In the risk society (Beck 1992) parents increasingly identify the world outside the home as one which their children must be shielded and in relation to which they must devise strategies of risk reduction

(James et al, 1998, p 7)

Discourses that have emphasised safeguarding and child protection in recent years have minimised children's exposure to risk. It is interesting that childhood was not always conceptualised in this way; in the 1800s young children worked in the factories and coal mines and suffered injuries and death from exposure to risk. Discourses around safeguarding are relatively recent, as are perspectives on agency. Historically, children were silenced and not given a voice, in stark contrast to current perspectives on childhood. As an early years practitioner, you have a legal duty to safeguard children and protect them from harm. However, eradicating risk from children's lives in the context of the early years setting is a dangerous move because children will encounter risk in their daily lives outside of the setting. Wrapping children up in cotton wool will not help them to assess, problem-solve or negotiate risk. Children need to be resilient to a range of risks and they need to be able to manage and negotiate risk. Children also need to take risks in their learning and experience 'failure', learn from it and recover. This will support their subsequent learning and development. Children need to be able to try out challenging tasks and not be worried about getting things wrong.

Exposing children to 'safe risk' is a useful way of developing their resilience. 'Safe risk' does not put children in danger but allows children to problem-solve and manage risk.

CRITICAL QUESTIONS

+ How can risk be integrated into outdoor learning?

+ Have safeguarding and child protection policies wrapped children up in cotton wool by providing them with safe, sterile and risk-free environments?

+ Why is exposure to risk important in children's lives?

Research by Tovey (2010) found that risky play provides children with opportunities to develop decision-making skills and assess risks. Tovey found that through engaging in risky play, children may sometimes succeed and sometimes fail. Failures, however, can enable children to learn from their mistakes and approach things differently in the future. Tovey argued that in today's increasingly regulated and controlled society, safety concerns have resulted in reduced opportunities for risky play.

CASE STUDY

A nursery provided the children with a weekly outdoor learning session in the local woods. The children walked to the woods in all weathers and participated in a range of activities. These included using branches, logs, fabric sheeting and other natural materials to create dens. The children played on the rope swing that was attached to a tree. They walked through the river in the woods and examined the wildlife in the river. They climbed trees and they walked across uneven ground. The wood was used as an opportunity for children to learn about habitats, animals and plants and about mathematics. The children collected branches to make different types of triangles, rectangles, squares, pentagons, hexagons and octagons. The children re-enacted stories in the wood and they explored the mini-beasts that lived under the logs.

ADVERSE CHILDHOOD EXPERIENCES

Adverse childhood experiences include stressors such as poverty, abuse, neglect, being in care or family breakdown, loss, family violence and responsibilities of care (Roffey, 2016). Research demonstrates that stressful and negative life circumstances impact detrimentally on self-worth, concentration, attendance, behaviour and mental health, all of which will affect children's learning and development across all areas (Mani et al, 2013). It has also been argued that long-term stressors are more damaging to mental health than acute, sudden events (Roffey, 2016). Research indicates, for example, that poverty is predictive of depression and anxiety (Fell and Hewstone, 2015). In addition, experiences of abuse and neglect can result in aggression, other forms of anti-social behaviour, poor self-worth and a wide range of mental health problems (Jutte et al, 2015). Psychological and behavioural disturbances are also associated with the experience of child sexual abuse (Roffey, 2016). Research demonstrates that children who experience domestic violence are more likely to be harmed themselves but are also at risk of multiple developmental problems (Roffey, 2016). Family breakdown can have a detrimental impact on children's learning and development and their mental health, although the way in which children experience family breakdown is dependent upon their age and how the breakdown is managed in the family (Dowling and Elliott, 2012).

Roffey has argued that *'when risks to wellbeing are chronic and on-going, resilience may need to be thought about differently'* (Roffey, 2017, p 2). Practitioners cannot simply expect children to 'get over' these adverse experiences. Many adverse childhood experiences can have long-term detrimental effects that extend well into adult life. Practitioners must recognise the factors that result in children's moods and behaviours and address these with sensitivity and empathy.

A national survey in England in 2013 revealed that 48 per cent of adults (aged 18–69) have experienced at least one adverse childhood experience, with 9 per cent experiencing four or more adverse childhood experiences over their childhood.

(www.aces.me.uk/files/2215/3495/0307/REACh_Evaluation_Report.pdf)

Bronfenbrenner's bioecological systems theory (Bronfenbrenner, 1979) has been influential in understanding the influences on childhood development. It positions the child within the following systems, all of which influence development.

+ Microsystem: these are contexts that directly impact the child's development, including family, the educational setting, religious institutions, peers and the community.

+ Mesosystem: these are the interconnections between the microsystems, such as the interactions that take place between parents and practitioners.

+ Macrosystem: the macrosystem describes the cultural contexts (or societal norms) that shape children's lives.

Other systems are identified in Bronfenbrenner's model but are not covered here. Adverse circumstances could have their origins in one or more of these systems. The model helps us to recognise the interconnectedness of different elements in the child's life. For example, if there is breakdown in the relationship between the child and their primary carer, this is an adverse circumstance that occurs in the microsystem. Other elements of the microsystem can attempt to counteract this negative experience; for example, through early years practitioners establishing strong, positive relationships with the child.

However, although this can reduce the effects of the adverse experience, it is not sufficient to compensate for the breakdown of the relationship between the child and their primary carer and this can have long-lasting effects that extend into adulthood.

- 93,000 children live in care;
- 24,300 children are in need of protection from neglect;
- 1 in 20 children experience sexual abuse;
- 50,000 children are in need of protection from abuse;
- 42 per cent of marriages end in divorce;
- it is estimated that 130,000 children live in homes with a high risk of domestic violence.

(Roffey, 2016)

CRITICAL QUESTIONS

+ To what extent have we created a 'cotton wool' society for children by removing their exposure to risk?
+ How can this affect children's resilience?

WHAT IS RESILIENCE?

It has been argued that *'children do not achieve resilience by their own efforts in "pulling themselves together"'* (Roffey, 2016, p 33). Their resilience is affected by the social contexts in which they are situated. The support of families, practitioners, community and religious organisations can help children to be resilient and cope better with adversity. According to Doll, *'resilience is a characteristic that emerges out of the systemic interdependence of children with their families, communities and schools'* (Doll, 2013, p 400). Resilience is a complex, multifaceted and dynamic construct. For example, some children may be resilient learners but not resilient in social situations or vice versa.

Although social context can influence resilience, so too can individual factors. For example, children with high levels of intelligence might be more able to rationalise their experiences, thus enabling them to cope better during times of adversity. Children who are confident are more likely to be able to talk about how they feel and how adverse experiences are affecting them. Talking about their experiences can help to develop resilience. However, it has been argued that confidence requires a context in which mistakes are accepted (Roffey, 2016) and as an individual characteristic it is therefore influenced by the social context in the child is positioned.

Young children need to be resilient in their learning so that when faced with challenging or unfamiliar tasks they do not simply give up. Resilience enables them to persevere with tasks in order to achieve mastery. They also need to learn to be resilient in social interactions when developing social relationships. Children need to learn to resolve conflicts, and practitioners play a critical role in enabling children to talk through conflicts. They need to learn that situations will arise within friendships that result in disagreements. Social resilience will enable children to resolve disputes so that friendships can be maintained. Children need to develop physical resilience during tasks that are designed to develop their gross and fine motor skills; for example, demonstrating stamina during physical activity. They also need to demonstrate emotional resilience by managing their own feelings and emotions in various situations.

These examples illustrate that resilience is not straightforward. Children can demonstrate resilience in one aspect but lack resilience in another aspect. As a practitioner, your role is to observe children in a range of contexts so that you can identify which aspects of resilience require further development.

Rutter (1987, p 317) argued that *'resilience is concerned with individual variations in response to risk. Some people succumb to stress and adversity whereas others overcome life hazards'*. Rutter also argued that resilience is not a fixed attribute, in that the same people who react adversely to a particular life stressor might cope well with the same stressor at another point in time. Therefore, resilience in relation to a specific stressor is not static and can be enhanced or weakened.

Bonnet and Bernard (2012) identify three aspects of resilience:

+ resilience is seen as an emotional reaction when faced with problematic or stressful situations;

+ the ability to calm down from a difficult situation within a realistic time frame;

+ the capacity to recover and continue with what they were doing before the stressor.

Taket et al (2012, p 39) argue that *'resilience is more appropriately conceived of as a human capacity that can be developed and strengthened in all people'.*

These perspectives all focus on an individual's ability to 'bounce-back' from a negative experience but while this is important, recovering from an experience is only one aspect of resilience. Resilient individuals are able to acknowledge how they feel. They are confident in knowing how and where to seek help by talking to others or seeking other forms of support. As an early years practitioner, you play a critical role in helping children to talk to adults about how they are feeling. Adults will interpret situations differently to children, so what a child may find stressful, an adult may not. It is important to acknowledge how children are feeling and to demonstrate empathy, even if the situation that results in the stress or anxiety appears to you to be relatively minor. If very young children (for example, babies) or children with special educational needs have not developed verbal communication, you will need to observe them to ascertain how they are feeling.

CRITICAL QUESTIONS

+ How does autism affect children's social and emotional resilience?
+ How can practitioners model the skill of resilience to children?

DEVELOPING RESILIENCE IN THE EARLY YEARS

It has been argued that although some protective factors are within the child, many are located within the social environment in which individuals live and learn (Roffey, 2017). This has significant implications for you as an early years practitioner in relation to your role in developing resilience in children.

Establishing warm, positive, trusting and supportive relationships is critical to enable children to become more resilient (Roffey, 2016). Roffey argues that *'for children to thrive they need at least one person who they can trust, thinks they are worthwhile and lets them know that they are lovable and capable'* (Roffey, 2016, p 34). As Bronfenbrenner says, *'In order to develop, a child needs the enduring, irrational involvement of one or more adults in care and joint activity with the child. Somebody has to be crazy about that kid'* (2005, p 262). The key worker plays a critical role in developing children's confidence and self-worth and these factors will impact positively on their ability to be resilient in a range of situations. As a practitioner, you play a crucial role in teaching children to persist and learn from their mistakes when they experience 'failure'. You should emphasise to children that making mistakes is a normal part of learning and children should not be afraid to try things, make mistakes and learn from this experience.

Experiencing a *'sense of connectedness'* or belonging to the setting is a recognised protective factor for mental health (DfE, 2015). Children need to feel included in the setting, and establishing friendships will facilitate a sense of belonging. After all, social connection is essential for optimal development (Roffey, 2017). You should support children to develop multiple friendships through giving them opportunities to socially interact and collaborate. Play-based learning is an effective tool for facilitating social interactions and enables children to learn in a variety of contexts. As a practitioner you will model appropriate social behaviours, including demonstrating respect, kindness and empathy towards others. These behaviours may not have been modelled in the home, but as children learn to understand the rules of positive social interactions they will be able to develop positive and long-lasting friendships.

The following factors will aid the development of resilience:

+ inclusive belonging and connectedness to the setting;

+ a strengths- and solutions-based approach;

+ high levels of social capital across the setting rooted in positive social values, such as kindness, trust, respect, fairness and acknowledgement;

+ high-quality interactions between children and practitioners;

+ positive peer relationships;

+ an emphasis on social and emotional learning.

(Roffey, 2017)

If these are embedded within the setting, children will develop confidence, self-worth and resilience. A strengths- and solutions-based approach focuses on practitioners demonstrating to children what they know and can do, thus providing positive acknowledgement of their abilities and character traits. Some children will arrive in the setting with feelings of low self-worth. Your role as a practitioner is to help children to recognise their strengths rather than their weaknesses. If children start thinking from a position of strength, they are more likely to try new activities and take risks in their learning. If they experience feelings of low self-worth they are less likely to be resilient to new challenges. The explicit modelling of the skills of social interaction and emotional regulation in both adult-directed tasks and through adult interactions in child-initiated play will support children. They will develop the skills they need to form positive social relationships with others and enable them to regulate their own feelings. It has been argued that the direct teaching of social and emotional skills supports the development of positive mental health in children (Durlak et al, 2011).

Providing children with agency increases both confidence and a sense of responsibility (Dobia et al, 2014). Children who are more confident and have a sense of responsibility are more likely to be resilient. Play-based learning provides a crucial vehicle for providing children with agency because it enables them to initiate their own learning. Additionally, providing children with regular opportunities to talk about how they feel and to identify from their perspective their strengths and areas for development allows them to have a voice. This builds confidence and in turn this will support the development of resilience.

CRITICAL QUESTIONS

+ While the Early Years Foundation Stage framework emphasises a strengths-based approach, it could be argued that the Early Learning Goals promote a deficit approach. To what extent do you agree with this argument?

+ How can you promote inclusion within your setting?

CASE STUDY

A range of problem-solving tasks were planned to develop the children's resilience in a nursery. In one task the children were asked to design a bridge using paper and card that was strong enough to support the weight of the three goats in The Three Billy Goats Gruff. They explored different ways of strengthening the material using folding techniques, including corrugation.

SUMMARY

This chapter discussed the overarching principles of the Early Years Foundation Stage framework and demonstrates how these reflect current discourses on childhood. It highlights how perspectives on childhood have changed significantly over time and it illustrates how discourses on childhood have shaped perspectives on resilience. The impact of adverse childhood experiences is presented within the context of children's resilience and the tensions associated with resilience are explored. The chapter also suggests some strategies for developing resilience in the early years setting.

CHECKLIST

This chapter has addressed:

✓ the concept of resilience;

✓ the changing perspectives on childhood and resilience;

✓ the impact of adverse childhood experiences on children's resilience;

✓ the approaches to developing resilience within the early years setting.

FURTHER READING

Robinson, M (2014) *The Feeling Child: Laying the Foundations of Confidence and Resilience (Foundations of Child Development).* Oxon: Routledge.

✚ CHAPTER 4

WORKING IN PARTNERSHIP TO ADDRESS NEEDS

PROFESSIONAL LINKS

This chapter addresses the following:

@ The Early Years Foundation Stage framework (DfE, 2017) emphasises the importance of working in partnership with parents and other professionals.

@ The Special Educational Needs and Disability Code of Practice (DfE and DoH, 2015) emphasises the importance of working in partnership with parents, external agencies and the child in addressing the child's needs.

CHAPTER OBJECTIVES

By the end of this chapter you will understand:

+ the importance of working in partnership in the early years;

+ the barriers to effective partnership working in the early years;

+ the important contribution of communities of practice to effective partnership working;

+ strategies to facilitate partnership working in the early years.

INTRODUCTION

This chapter addresses the importance of working in partnership to support young children's mental health. Throughout this chapter the term 'parent' has been used to refer to parents and legal guardians of the child. In this chapter you will learn about the importance of working in partnership with parents, children and external services to support children's mental health needs. You will also be introduced to some strategies for facilitating these partnerships in the early years. Some of the professional challenges associated with partnership working and ways of overcoming these are addressed.

As an early years practitioner, you will understand the importance of children's holistic development. If children are not mentally healthy then it is more difficult for them to learn. You will already be aware of the critical link between children's behaviour and their learning, but you might be less aware of the link between their mental health and their progress across all other areas of learning.

Effective social and emotional environments in the early years promote positive well-being in children. The causes of mental ill-health in children are complex and multifaceted. Effective partnership working will enable you to address some of the many risk factors that can have a detrimental impact on children's mental well-being. Social care services are well placed to address family factors that might result in mental ill-health. Health care professionals are best able to provide interventions to address health-related factors that arise from mental ill-health. As a practitioner, you play a critical role in developing effective partnerships with parents and children, although it is not always easy to achieve this. This chapter provides examples of how you might develop positive partnerships and advice on when to refer children to external services.

WORKING WITH PARENTS AND CARERS

Parents are children's first educators. They know the child best and have valuable insights that they can offer to practitioners. Effective parental partnerships in early years settings have a positive impact on outcomes for children (Hill and Taylor, 2004). The Early Years Foundation Stage framework (EYFS framework) highlights the role of practitioners in developing partnerships with parents. The Special Educational Needs and Disability (SEND) Code of Practice (DfE and DoH, 2015) emphasises the importance of working in partnership with parents during the process of identifying children's needs. Parents will have observed their child's mood and behaviour in a range of contexts and should be able to support you in your assessment of need(s). Any assessment by practitioners can therefore only be a partial assessment of the child based on your observations within the setting. You will also need to develop effective relationships with grandparents and other family members if you have more contact with the wider family on a daily basis.

If you suspect that a child in your setting has a mental health need then you will need to carry out observations of the child in a range of contexts. These may include observations of the child when they are engaged in both indoor and outdoor learning. You should also observe the child during participation in child-initiated independent learning, child-initiated adult-supported learning and adult-directed learning. You will also need to observe the child when they are learning individually and during participation in collaborative tasks. During these observations you will be trying to ascertain whether the child's mental health needs are triggered within a specific context or whether the needs are evident across a range of contexts. You will also need to observe the child across a time duration to identify whether the need is temporary or potentially more serious.

Your observations can be supported through parents' own observations of the child's mood and behaviour outside of the setting. The following guidance offers a useful way of framing an initial conversation with the parent.

+ *'In the setting I have noticed that X appears to be [withdrawn/sad/ angry/anxious, etc].'*

+ *'Have you observed this also outside of the setting?'*

+ *'Can you suggest any reasons why X is demonstrating these behaviours?'*

+ *'I have noticed that the trigger might be...'*

+ *'Have you also noticed this at home?'*

+ *'How do you manage this at home?'*

+ *'Let's talk about how we can support X.'*

It is critical that you keep an open mind and do not judge the parent. Your role is not to blame the parent for the child's difficulties but to work together with the parent to identify solutions for the child.

It is also important to bear in mind that parents of children with mental health needs may also have poor mental health. Parents who are experiencing mental ill-health are not well-placed to support their child's mental health. You play an important role in signposting these parents to external sources of support within the community so that parents who experience mental ill-health can get the support they need. Some settings are also adopting more proactive approaches to supporting parents and the case study that follows illustrates one such strategy.

CASE STUDY

An early years setting was situated in an area of social deprivation in the north of England. Many of the parents were unemployed and were experiencing financial difficulties. Some of them were struggling to pay their household bills on time and buy food for their family. There were those who faced eviction due to non-payment of rent and the threat of homelessness. Many of the parents appeared to be stressed, depressed or anxious or a combination of all three.

The manager of the setting decided to organise a series of workshops for parents to support them with simple financial management. All parents were invited to participate in the workshops and refreshments were provided. Sessions included:

+ how to manage on a tight budget;

+ shopping smartly;

+ managing stress, anxiety and depression;

+ services in the community that can offer support;

+ parents as role models;

+ mindfulness.

Attendance at the sessions was good and evaluations of the workshops were extremely positive. Follow-up sessions were organised to help parents to recognise the signs of mental ill-health in their children. Parents were introduced to the signs and symptoms of mental ill-health and provided with simple techniques to support their child to manage stress, anxiety and depression. Parents were introduced to the importance of physical activity and social connectivity in supporting positive mental health for both children and adults. They were also taught about the important role that volunteering can play in promoting positive mental health. Above all, the sessions had a positive impact on parents' perceptions of mental health. They had started to talk openly to others about their own mental health and their own mental health literacy improved.

INVOLVING PARENTS IN PLANNING AND REVIEWING PROGRESS

Once initial mental health needs have been identified, your role as a practitioner is to work with parents to identify ways of supporting the child. It is important to review the child's progress regularly with parents and to decide on 'next steps' together, particularly in relation to decisions about interventions that can be implemented or whether to refer the child on to external services for additional support. Generally, parental consent will be necessary before a referral can take place.

During review meetings it is crucial to ascertain information about the child's mental health outside the context of the setting. This will help to identify whether the child's mental health is affected by a specific context and therefore this should aid the identification of triggers for mental ill-health.

CRITICAL QUESTIONS

+ How might you develop effective partnerships with parents who are resistant to mental health?

+ How might you work with parents who are unable to manage their own mental health so that positive outcomes can be achieved for the child?

43

- Approximately one in six adults in England reported experiencing a mental health problem in the past week.

- Over 2 million children are estimated to be living with a parent who has a common mental health disorder.

(www.nspcc.org.uk/preventing-abuse/child-protection-system/
parental-mental-health)

The Effective Provision of Pre-School Education (EPPE) research (Sylva et al, 2004) is a seminal research study into early years provision. The research found that:

+ what parents do with children at home makes a significant difference to young children's development;

+ when parents engage their child in a range of home learning activities, these serve as protective factors to children's social and emotional development;

+ examples of these activities include reading with the child, teaching songs and nursery rhymes, painting and drawing, playing with letters and numbers, visiting the library, teaching the alphabet and numbers, taking children on visits and creating regular opportunities for them to play with their friends at home;

+ these activities were all associated with higher intellectual and social/ behavioural scores;

+ the home learning environment was only moderately associated with parents' educational or occupational level, so what parents do with their children is more important than who the parents are.

WORKING WITH HEALTH CARE PROFESSIONALS

Health care professionals play a crucial role in supporting children's development, including their mental health, in the very early stages of their development. All children in England must undertake a 'progress check' at the age of two to identify whether their development is age-appropriate. These progress checks are conducted by practitioners and mental health needs will usually be identified through assessment of children's personal, social and emotional development.

All early years settings are required to work in partnership with health care professionals who can support children's development. These include nurses and doctors. Doctors can identify whether a child has a diagnosable mental health need and nurses can provide guidance on how to manage specific conditions including stress, anxiety, depression and self-harm. The general principle is that parental consent should be sought before children are referred to health care services.

Nurses can play an important role in facilitating professional learning for staff within the setting. They can lead professional training on how to identify the signs and symptoms of mental ill-health and they can work with specific children within the context of the setting to provide the intervention they need.

WORKING WITH SOCIAL CARE PROFESSIONALS

Some children who display signs of mental ill-health will also be living in families and communities that place them at risk of harm. Children who experience abuse and neglect are more likely to demonstrate signs of mental ill-health. Children who are exposed to family conflict, including domestic violence, are also at greater risk of mental ill-health. Children who do not feel loved or cared for, or those who have not developed secure attachments with a primary caregiver, are at increased risk of developing mental ill-health (Bowlby, 2012; National Institute for Health and Care Excellence, 2016). Children from areas of social deprivation are more significantly at risk of developing poor mental health.

While it is important not to stereotype types of families and communities, it is, nevertheless, important to be aware of the risk factors. If you suspect that a child is at risk of, or is experiencing, neglect, physical, sexual or psychological abuse, then you have a duty to report this to the designated safeguarding leader within the setting. This case will then be picked up through the safeguarding processes that have been developed to meet the statutory safeguarding requirements.

CRITICAL QUESTIONS

+ What are the challenges associated with partnership working?

+ How might you overcome these?

WORKING WITH CHILD AND ADOLESCENT MENTAL HEALTH SERVICES

Child and Adolescent Mental Health Services (CAMHS) is a branch of the National Health Service that exists to support children and young people with the most severe mental health needs. The service is made up of health professionals, including counsellors, clinical psychologists, support workers and therapists. Children who are referred to CAMHS have needs that are so severe that they cannot be addressed in the setting or the home. They are used when specialist support is required to help the child to manage their mental health. Services have lengthy waiting lists and referral criteria are strict. This means that not all children successfully secure a referral to access these specialist services.

WHEN TO REFER?

You will need to check the referral criteria of your local CAMHS service. However generally the criteria for referral are that the need(s) must be:

+ severe;

+ complex – this means that there may be multiple risk factors that are present, and the child may be experiencing complex family problems;

+ enduring – usually CAMHS services will not admit children who have demonstrated a mental illness for less than three months.

You will need to support the referral with documentary evidence of your assessments. These should include observations of the child in varying contexts and, where appropriate, progress checks against identified milestones. You will also need to include assessments over a duration of time to demonstrate whether a need is increasing in severity.

CRITICAL QUESTIONS

+ Do you agree that a mental health need should be 'complex' to gain a referral to CAMHS? Explain your answer.

+ Do you agree that a mental health need should be enduring? Explain your answer.

+ What are the warning signs that may indicate that an infant may have mental ill-health?

Rates of mental disorders increase with age: 5.5 per cent of 2–4 year-old children experienced a mental disorder in 2017, compared to 16.9 per cent of 17–19 year-olds.

(https://digital.nhs.uk/data-and-information/publications/statistical/
mental-health-of-children-and-young-people-in-england/2017/2017)

Lave and Wenger (1991) developed the idea of *'communities of practice'*. A community of practice is characterised by the following.

+ Domain: this is the area of knowledge that brings the group together. All members of the group share an interest in the domain and have expertise in it, which they wish to share across the group.

+ Community: a strong sense of community is essential for effective multi-agency collaboration. The community is united by its sense of purpose and commitment to the domain.

+ Practice: while knowledge is essential, communities of practice exist to develop practices and share these across the group.

Thus, multi-agency teams are communities of practice that exist to support the needs of the child. The multi-agency team may include education practitioners and health and social care practitioners. It should also include the parents and the child. Within this team everyone is able to bring their own unique and sometimes specialised knowledge to the community. Parents are experts in their child and children are also experts in their own lives. Practitioners from education, health and social care also have their own disciplinary knowledge from which the community can benefit.

A strong sense of community within a community of practice is essential. It is therefore important to respect the different roles of people within the team and to value the distinct contribution that different people can make to the community. It is crucial that everyone understands the roles and responsibilities of all community members and the limits to these roles. It is important to take account of professional boundaries and to trust that all members of the community will act honestly and with integrity.

It is important to develop a shared language to facilitate communication between different members of a community of practice. Heath, social care and education all have their own language, and professional jargon associated with specific disciplines can form a barrier to effective communication. The use of acronyms and discipline-specific terminology should be avoided where possible because it can be alienating. It is also important to communicate effectively with parents by avoiding the overuse of professional jargon.

Developing a community of practice that functions effectively can be challenging. Logistical problems might make it difficult for the community to meet together in person. Each discipline may have its own ethical code, which means that information cannot always be shared across the team. This can cause frustration for other community members. Additionally, each service will be managing significant caseloads, and this can delay the speed at which information is shared.

In recent years several high-profile cases of child deaths have gained media publicity due to ineffective multi-agency collaboration. Reviews of these cases have identified several recurrent factors that resulted in the death of the child. These include:

+ not sharing information or sharing information too late;

+ inconsistent record-keeping;

+ lack of effective communication between different agencies.

SHARING INFORMATION

Data protection legislation should not be a barrier to sharing information in cases where young people are at risk of harm. If you need to share information about a child, where possible you should explain to children why you need to share information, what information will be shared and who the information will be shared with. It is better to get the child's consent, but if you believe that a child is at risk you are still able to share the information.

According to HM Government (2018), information that is shared should be:

+ proportionate: only share the information that is necessary by ensuring that information shared is proportionate to the need to share it and to the potential risks to the child;

+ relevant: only share relevant information;

+ adequate: ensure that the information is adequate and enables other professionals to fulfil their professional commitments;

+ accurate: ensure that the information is accurate and includes facts, not opinions;

+ timely: information should be shared in a timely way, particularly in cases where the child is at risk or in immediate danger;

+ secure: follow the school's policy to ensure that information is stored securely.

When sharing information, you will need to ensure that you are compliant with the new data protection regulations (General Data Protection Regulations, GDPR) which affect all organisations, including schools and early years settings.

CASE STUDY

An early years setting in the south of England wanted to focus on developing partnerships with children. Hannah, a practitioner who had worked at the nursery for 18 months, created a 'feelings' board that included photographs and names of each child. At the start of each day the children selected a 'feelings' card and matched it to their name. The cards depicted a range of different feelings including happiness, sadness, anger and mixed feelings. The children quickly adapted to this routine. Each day Hannah identified the children who had selected negative feelings and held a conversation with them. The aim of this was to provide the children with an opportunity to talk about their feelings, to identify why they had those feelings and what steps might be taken to change the negative feelings into positive feelings.

The children enjoyed selecting the feelings card and there was no evidence that children were reluctant to select the negative feelings cards. After several weeks Hannah identified a group of children to be well-being champions. These children were taught how to support other children who had identified that they did not feel happy. They were taught how to do 'kind things' for these children, which included:

+ inviting them into their play;

+ talking to them about how they feel;

+ offering to play with them at playtime;

+ offering to sit with them at lunchtime.

This strategy was very successful because the champions were empowered by the role. They enjoyed helping their peers and it made them feel important.

CRITICAL QUESTIONS

+ How might you select the well-being champions?

+ How might you monitor the impact of this initiative?

+ What barriers might you have to overcome if you implemented this approach and how would you address these?

SUMMARY

This chapter has emphasised the importance of working effectively in partnership with parents, external services and the child to support children's mental health needs. You have been prompted to consider the challenges associate with partnership working and ways of overcoming these. Through the case studies you have been introduced to examples of effective practice in the early years. The chapter has highlighted the risks associated with ineffective multi-agency collaboration. It has emphasised the need for different professional service teams to develop mutual respect and a shared language to aid communication between members of a community of practice.

CHECKLIST

This chapter has addressed:

✓ the key partners that can support you to address mental ill-health in children;

✓ ways of working in partnership with parents;

✓ ways of working in partnership with the child;

✓ referrals to health and social care services.

FURTHER READING

Anning, A, Cottrell, D, Frost, N, Green, J and Robinson, M (2006) *Developing Multiprofessional Teamwork For Integrated Children's Services: Research, Policy and Practice.* Milton Keynes: Open University Press.

Gasper, M (2010) *Multi-Agency Working in the Early Years: Challenges and Opportunities.* London: Sage.

✚ CHAPTER 5

THE IMPORTANCE OF SELF-REGULATION IN THE EARLY YEARS

PROFESSIONAL LINKS

This chapter addresses the following:

- Department for Education (2017) *Statutory Framework for the Early Years Foundation Stage: Setting the Standards for Learning, Development and Care for Children from Birth to Five*. London: DfE.

- The Early Years Foundation Stage has three prime areas of learning (section 1.5). Two of these areas are particularly relevant to this chapter:

  communication and language, which involves giving children opportunities to develop their confidence and skills in expressing themselves; and to speak and listen in a range of situations;

personal, social and emotional development, which involves helping children to develop a positive sense of themselves and others, to form positive relationships and develop respect for others, to develop social skills and learn how to manage their feelings, to understand appropriate behaviour in groups, and to have confidence in their own abilities.

CHAPTER OBJECTIVES

By the end of this chapter you will understand:

+ the relationship between self-regulation, school readiness and mental health;

+ how to develop self-regulation and related skills in young children.

INTRODUCTION

The EYFS (DfE, 2017) promotes teaching and learning to ensure children's 'school readiness' (p 5), but there are different interpretations as to what school readiness actually means; the question arises about what it actually is that children are getting ready for. Some early years settings and parents interpret school readiness formally, perceiving it to include sitting still for periods of time, following instructions, recognising numbers and letters, reading and writing, and therefore preparing children for the expectations of school. This chapter explores the importance of self-regulation to the development of school readiness, rather than academic capabilities.

Self-regulation and executive function skills underlie many of the behaviours and attributes associated with successful school adjustment (Blair, 2002). Children have the potential to develop self-regulating skills through positive experiences, effective environments and affirmative relationships with adults. Early years practitioners can support children to self-regulate by providing a range of play opportunities that develop communication skills, negotiation, decision-making and taking others' perspectives into account (Kangas et al, 2015). This type of practice can help a child become socially competent, develop executive functioning and eventually be able to regulate their own behaviour, emotions and responses without adult support. Development of self-regulated behaviour is said to support well-being and success at school more powerfully that early academic content (Bingham and Whitebread, 2012).

Social and emotional skill development is vital to children's well-being and mental health (Goodman et al, 2015) and mental ill-health in childhood is linked to poorer educational attainment and negative outcomes later in life (Early Intervention Foundation, 2017).

SELF-REGULATION AND EXECUTIVE FUNCTION DEVELOPMENT

Bodrova and Leong (2015) suggest self-regulation has two sides: the first is the ability to control impulses and to *stop doing something* and the second involves being able to *do something* as required, such as take turns or follow instructions.

Goodman et al (2015) place self-regulation alongside self-control when outlining the five groupings of social and emotional skills in children and define it as being *'how children manage and express emotions, and the extent to which they overcome short-term impulsivity in order to pri-oritise higher pursuits'* (p 7). The ability to self-regulate in the early years is closely related to school readiness and is said to predict school achievement better than IQ scores (Blair 2002; Blair and Razza, 2007). Blair and Raver (2015) explain that self-regulation develops from infancy onwards, it facilitates effective early learning, but the environment has a key role to play in this development.

As children learn to self-regulate they become more able to manage their feelings, concentrate and share. They begin to depend on their own self-control rather than adult regulation. Thus, they are *'"masters of their own behaviour" rather than "slaves to the environment"'* (Bodrova and Leong, 2015, p 374). Executive function development also begins in infancy, is shaped by experience and draws on self-regulatory skills, enabling children to develop:

+ *working memory, the ability to hold information and use it;*

+ *inhibitory control, master impulses to resist distractions and think before acting;*

+ *flexible thinking, able to adjust to changing demands.*

(Center on the Developing Child at Harvard University, 2014)

Day-to-day experience in an effective early years setting can encourage social and emotional skill development, which in turn supports future readiness for moving into school. This help is particularly important when a child may be living in poverty or in other difficult circumstances, where structure may be absent from their lives at home. Children experiencing adverse life conditions are more likely to be at a developmental disadvantage and present difficult behaviour as a result of poor self-regulatory skills. Blair and Raver (2015) suggest that such disadvantage can be turned around by appropriate structured experiences. Bodrova and Leong (2008) suggest play activities in which children set, negotiate and follow the rules are important to self-regulation. Early years practitioners who understand when a child may be unable to regulate their behaviour and is not simply 'acting out', are well placed to offer practical, supportive and age-appropriate strategies.

INFANTS

Infants are exposed to a series of new and different experiences involving people, movement and sounds; they are dependent on safe, caring adults who are in tune with their needs to regulate their responses. Bridges and Grolnick (1995) suggest that distraction and soothing strategies carried out by an attentive caregiver offers co-regulation and the child is guided to increasingly perform such strategies for themselves. These include the following.

+ When a baby awakens and becomes upset to find they are alone, if the adult responds quickly with reassurance then the baby will be comforted and become calm; this strategy encourages self-soothing.

+ An infant who is distressed by something new or a sudden noise can be pacified by the attention of an adult who uses distraction to draw the child's attention to something more pleasant and interesting. Adult response and quick calming helps infants learn to calm and distract themselves.

+ Self-regulatory development can be observed when babies respond to simple commands such as a 'no' gesture when faced with the temptation of touching something prohibited.

TODDLERS: 1–2 YEARS

At this point in early childhood children are beginning to develop independence and self-awareness. From around the age of one year, children want to be self-reliant and they wish to attempt tasks for themselves. This can be a difficult time for them, especially if they are unable to achieve their goal or if they are prevented from doing so by the carer. Placing constraints on children can lead to tears and anger.

It can be a frustrating time for the child and challenging for the adult, but it is reassuring to know that, rather than being deliberately awkward or badly behaved, the child is experiencing a stage of development, learning to self-regulate and become independent. Calm and supportive adults can help these young children to manage irritability and reduce the stress and anxiety they may be experiencing. This stage of development is best served if the adult offers appropriate solutions, or better still distracts to avoid possible disturbance. Useful strategies are outlined below.

+ Children can sometimes find it hard to complete tasks when required, so it can help to offer choices. For example, if a toddler is reluctant to put on a coat to play outside, they may respond better to *'left arm first or right arm?'*

+ This age-group may enjoy imitating actions and songs with gestures encourage memory, waiting and recall.

+ Games with simple rules can be introduced – such as taking turns to throw beanbags into a box or roll a ball down a tube.

+ Adults who are attentive and in tune with a young child's needs are on hand to guide and help manage emotions.

3–5 YEAR-OLDS

At this stage children:

+ use the term 'taking turns' rather than 'sharing' – this is more tangible to young children;

+ struggle with instructions such as tidying up when engrossed in a game or activity so you could try give them the heads-up *'tidy up time in ten minutes'* then *'five minutes left before we...'* Children may not at first understand how long that gives them, but a grasp of time does begin to form.

Practitioners can:

+ use everyday situations to develop impulse control; for example, while children are waiting for turns to participate in an activity, create another activity that has to be carried out beforehand;

+ use timers: some activities lend themselves to being timed and setting a timer gives children a real-time cue to help them wait and control their immediate impulse;

+ acknowledge the challenge, for example by saying *'it can be hard to wait can't it? Why not do something else while you are waiting?'*, and have a suggestion of what they can do;

+ give children plenty of opportunities to exercise choice; this is helpful as it develops decision-making skills and gives a sense of accomplishment;

+ support children to make more complex decisions that involve more options;

+ play simple games such as musical statues;

+ practise silence – listen to the sounds in the building or better still when outside the building, such as the sounds of traffic or birds.

An important and effective strategy for all age groups is for adults to model self-regulation. One example of modelling is to show children how to persevere with a frustrating task without getting upset. Talking to the children about how difficult the task was also helps, for example *'Phew that was hard... good job I didn't get upset, I might not have been able to finish it if I had.'*

CRITICAL QUESTIONS

+ Consider how the strategies above link to and support self-regulation.

+ Which strategies do you think are most helpful in preparation for school experience and why?

The State of Education Survey identifies that 31 per cent of primary school leaders say that more than half of new pupils are not school-ready.

——————

(The Key, 2016)

PLAYFUL LEARNING AND ITS ROLE IN SELF-REGULATION AND CHILDREN'S WELL-BEING

Section 1.8 of the EYFS framework identifies the significance of play to children's development and recommends that areas of learning and development are to be addressed through *'planned, purposeful play'* with a mixture of *'adult-led and child-initiated activity'* (DfE, 2017, p 9).

Whitebread (2012, p 9) reminds us that play and its role in well-being has been valued throughout history, from the classical societies of ancient Greece and Rome, through medieval Europe and into more contemporary times. Play-based learning is well supported by current researchers as the most appropriate approach to development and learning in the early years. According to Zosh et al (2017, p 32): *'the evidence on learning through play is mounting; more than an enjoyable experience, engaging with the world in playful ways is essential for laying a foundation for learning early in life'*. Play is well documented as supporting social and emotional development and there is a growing body of evidence that shows that experiences during early childhood can have lifelong consequences for health and well-being (Moore and Lynch 2017; Zosh et al, 2017), thus supporting the skills needed for adulthood in the twenty-first century (Hirsch-Pasek et al, 2016).

Gray (2011) reminds us that play supports development functions that promote children's mental health (p 458) and in social play children learn to regulate their emotions because *'cooperation and conflict'* is involved (p 456). When engaged in playful experiences, children are learning how to make decisions, solve problems, develop self-control and follow rules. Those skills are all related to self-regulation and inform the type of playful activities that practitioners can provide for children from a very young age. Through play children can:

+ make decisions – offering choices of toys, outfits and books;

+ solve problems – posting shapes, puzzles, simple jigsaws and even self-feeding;

+ develop self-control – taking turns, waiting (in the case of babies, this would be while being distracted);

+ follow rules – simple action songs.

The practitioner can offer more complexity as the child grows, but it can be helpful to remember that self-control and following rules can be part of everyday activities in the setting. Steiner Waldorf settings promote rhythm and repetition, believing regular patterns and routines in the day not only offer a sense of security, but develop self-confidence, memory, and remove the need for *'constant direction and instruction'* (House, 2011, p 183) thus helping children to acquire self-management skills.

In the first stages of play, children are most involved in exploring objects. As a child grows their play evolves, becoming more sophisticated, drawing on additional skill development such as role-play and make-believe play.

when play is mature, children have defined roles and ... play scenarios that are complex and ... planned in advance.

(Bodrova and Leong, 2007)

Mature make-believe play offers an excellent opportunity to develop self-regulation skills because children are behaving to a set of actions defined by the role they are acting out. Home corners, shops and hospitals all play a part in this as they offer mechanisms to act out children's lived experiences.

In play a child is always above his average age, above his daily behavior; in play it is as though he were a head taller than himself.

(Vygotsky, 1967, p 16)

CASE STUDY

Holly was nearly four years old and had moved to a new nursery. David, one of the practitioners, was reading a story to the whole group in 'Poppies' room. Most of the children were listening and joining in with the repetitive lines of the story. Holly was distracted and eventually tried to walk off the mat, standing on the legs of other children as she did so. David realised it would be a battle to get Holly to sit down again so he lifted her off the mat, Holly immediately started to cry, wriggled out of his grasp and went to stand next to the wall.

Later, at the play-dough table, Holly was sitting quietly with one of the students on placement. When other children joined the table, Holly tried to gather all the play-dough away from them. The student tried to persuade Holly to share but she became upset and swept all the dough onto the floor.

During the team catch-up at the end of the day it was decided that Holly needed more support to control her emotions, adapt to new situations and the other children. Over the following days Holly's key worker, Jane, introduced self-regulatory play activities that involved simple turn-taking and sharing. Games such as matching pictures, were accompanied by conversation and explanation so Holly understood the rules and what was expected. At first the tasks involved just Jane and Holly but gradually the games involved other children. It was not too long before Holly's experiences at nursery became more positive and happier as she learned to control her emotions and play co-operatively with other children.

The Mental Health of Children and Young People in England report (NHS, 2017) examines the prevalence of mental health disorders in preschool children (2–4 year-olds) in England in 2017 and states that 1 in 18 (5.5 per cent) of pre-school children were identified with a mental disorder under the following groupings:

- emotional disorders;
- behavioural disorders;
- hyperactivity disorders.

POLICY AND PRACTICE TENSIONS

Section 1.8 of the EYFS framework draws attention to the fact that practitioners have to create a balance between activities led by children and those led by adults, that there is an *'ongoing judgement to be made'* (DfE, 2017, p 9).

Broadhead et al (2010) refer to such judgements as being a policy/practice tension between transmissive/directive (adult-led) and emergent/responsive (child-led) pedagogical approaches (p 15). Although the authors advocate an integrated approach, there is caution as to how the balance might be interpreted. There is concern among early years researchers that play, a vital aspect of a child's life and healthy development, is lacking the attention it requires in the pursuit of early learning.

Practitioners need to ensure play experiences are not formalised in a way that the same activities are set for all children simply as a device to record outcomes against the Early Learning Goals in the EYFS. Such practice would eventually eliminate opportunities for children to play, initiate play activities and develop a sense of ownership and self-efficacy (Whitebread, 2012, p 10).

Gray (2011) refers to the general decline of play for children over the second half of the twentieth century and draws attention to the increased time given to adult-directed activities and an increase in academically focused pre-schools. Bodrova and Leong (2008) also suggest that the decline in make-believe play is partly a result of increased adult-led learning and recreation.

CASE STUDY

Harry and George are happily playing together in the nursery. They are setting up the wood rail track, talking to each other as they plan the shape it will be. When they fetch the box of engines and carriages they start to disagree as they both want the blue engine. At first they argue and then start to push each other. George starts to cry and sits down on the floor. The practitioner who has been observing them wipes George's eyes then talks quietly to both of them about sharing and taking turns. The boys eventually smile at each other and return to their game, playing quite amicably for the rest of the time. This is a good example of self-regulation. Both boys were able to calm down, redirect their attention and control. This an example of self-soothing to deal with anxiety – an important life skill.

SUMMARY

This chapter has highlighted the importance of supporting children with social and emotional development, including self-regulation, with some appropriate strategies signposted. Embedding strategies into the setting is particularly beneficial for children from backgrounds of disadvantage as they may have weaker skills than their peers (Houghton et al, 2011). This chapter has emphasised the importance of playful activities to a young child's development. However, there is a cautious note that you are invited to consider. Through play children develop important life skills, confidence, control and positive self-image. By providing opportunities for playful learning, early years professionals play a hugely significant role in supporting children's mental health (Inness, 2015).

Overall this is a wide topic and although coverage is not exhaustive, this important and interesting area of early years pedagogy and practice is one that you can explore further using the examples of further reading.

CHECKLIST

This chapter has addressed:

✓ the importance of self-regulation to the healthy development of all young children;

✓ the role of play in social and emotional development;

✓ the need for caution required when interpreting the Early Learning Goals in the EYFS.

FURTHER READING

Video: *InBrief: Early Childhood Mental Health.* [online] Available at: https://developingchild.harvard.edu/resources/inbrief-early-childhood-mental-health (accessed 28 February 2019).

Bodrova, E and Leong, D J (2008) Developing Self-Regulation in Kindergarten: Can We Keep All the Crickets in the Basket? *Young Children*, 63: 56–58.

Center on the Developing Child at Harvard University (2014) *Enhancing and Practicing Executive Function Skills with Children from Infancy to Adolescence.* [online] Available at: www.developingchild.harvard.edu (accessed 28 February 2019).

+ CHAPTER 6

IDENTIFYING AND SUPPORTING EARLY YEARS CHILDREN WITH POSSIBLE MENTAL HEALTH NEEDS

PROFESSIONAL LINKS

This chapter addresses the following:

Department for Education (2017) *Statutory Framework for the Early Years Foundation Stage: Setting the Standards for Learning, Development and Care for Children from Birth to Five*. London: DfE.

CHAPTER OBJECTIVES

By the end of this chapter you will understand:

+ how to identify mental ill-health in the early years;

+ how to support children with specific mental health needs.

INTRODUCTION

This chapter introduces you to common types of mental ill-health in early childhood and provides some useful strategies that you can use to support children with specific needs. Children who are not mentally healthy are less likely to thrive. Their personal, social and emotional development is critical because it affects every other area of learning and development. A range of factors can affect children's mental health, including individual, community and family-related factors. Children's experiences in the setting can also influence their mental health. It is clear that mental illness does not just begin during adolescence. Many problems that are evident in children at the age of 14 are also evident during early childhood. Despite this, there is still a reluctance in society to accept that young children can demonstrate mental ill-health. This chapter begins by examining the aspects of personal, social and emotional development in the Early Years Foundation Stage framework (DfE, 2017) that can influence children's mental health. It then identifies some key warning signs of mental ill-health that practitioners may notice during their observations of children in a range of contexts. Finally, it examines common types of mental ill-health that children may experience in the early years.

PERSONAL, SOCIAL AND EMOTIONAL DEVELOPMENT

Personal, social and emotional development (PSED) is a prime area of learning in the early years. This is because it underpins all other areas of learning and development. It is the area of learning and development that relates most closely to mental health. Children's development in the specific areas will be affected by their development in PSED. If children lack self-confidence and self-awareness then this will affect their cognitive, physical, social and emotional development. If they find it difficult to establish relationships with others, this will impact detrimentally on their ability to learn with and from others. If they find it difficult to manage their feelings and behaviour and are unable to adjust their behaviour to fit the context of the setting, this will affect their ability to learn effectively.

SELF-CONFIDENCE AND SELF-AWARENESS

Children that are confident are able to try new activities and take risks. They are able to ask for help when they need it, select resources and learn from their mistakes. Children who lack self-confidence are generally less willing to try new activities and less willing to take risks and this limits their learning potential. They may become anxious and stressed when they are presented with new activities and experiences, and this can then prevent them from benefitting from new opportunities.

Some children may demonstrate signs of attachment disorder. They may have developed insecure, unstable or weak attachments with their primary carer. Consequently, they may feel rejected, unloved and neglected. These early experiences can have a detrimental effect on their confidence and this can result in feelings of anxiety when they are presented with unfamiliar tasks or experiences. As a practitioner you play a crucial role in supporting all children to develop self-confidence and self-awareness. Through establishing warm, trusting and positive relationships with children, you can support them to develop their self-confidence. You can gradually introduce children to new activities and experiences by initially scaffolding their learning to build their confidence. Once they gain confidence, they will be able to undertake tasks and experiences independently. You also play a critical role in teaching children to ask for help when they need it.

Vygotsky's Zone of Proximal Development (Vygotsky, 1978) refers to the distance between a learner's actual level of development and their potential level of development. This is the level that the learner is capable of reaching with the support of a more able other. Wood et al (1976) used the term 'scaffolding' to describe the support structures that need to be established to move the learner through their Zone of Proximal Development. Adult interaction in child-initiated play is a direct application of scaffolding a child through their Zone of Proximal Development.

MAKING RELATIONSHIPS

Learning in the early years is fundamentally a social process. Learning through play is critical for all aspects of a child's development. Collaborative learning enables children to learn the skills of negotiation, conflict resolution, regulation, problem-solving, empathy and risk-taking. In addition, collaborative play-based learning develops children's vocabulary, language and communication skills that underpin the development of their literacy skills. If children are not able to form relationships, then they miss out on the opportunities to develop these skills.

Some children will need greater support to help them to understand how to establish effective relationships. They may have been exposed to models of violent, manipulative, disrespectful and controlling relationships in the home. These children may need to be taught the skills that underpin the development of effective relationships. These include:

+ turn-taking and sharing;

+ conflict resolution;

+ demonstrating empathy;

+ listening to others;

+ respect for others.

Practitioners may need to model these skills through intervening in children's play. Through playing alongside children, you can model explicitly the skills that underpin the development of effective relationships. You can also read stories to children that address the theme of relationships and you can model positive relationships through your interactions with children and adults in the setting. For children who have not been exposed to positive relationships at home, these strategies will introduce them to models of appropriate relationships and support them in adjusting their behaviour when they are in the setting.

MANAGING FEELINGS AND BEHAVIOUR

Children should be encouraged to talk about their feelings. You may need to support them in developing their understanding of feelings by explicitly teaching them about different types of feelings. These include feeling happy, sad, worried, nervous, angry, jealous, excited and so on. Providing children with a 'feelings curriculum' will broaden their vocabulary and enable them to name their feelings. Stories that focus on different feelings are also a very effective way of teaching children about feelings. Essentially, children need to know that it is normal to experience negative feelings and that everyone experiences these from time to time. Your role as a practitioner is to provide them with some strategies to help them to manage their feelings. Children also need to be supported to recognise feelings in others and to show empathy. They need to be supported to follow simple rules in the setting, to adjust their behaviour in different contexts and to adapt to changes in routine. Enabling children to manage their own behaviour will help them to learn more effectively in the setting.

WARNING SIGNS

Sudden changes in the child's mood or behaviour could indicate that a child has a mental health need. However, it is important that you observe the child in a range of contexts to establish whether the problem has been 'triggered' by a specific context. It is also important to observe the child over a period of time to identify if the problem is persistent. Common signs of mental ill-health in children include:

+ changes in mood;

+ changes in behaviour;

+ physical signs;

+ soiling;

+ drawings that might indicate that the child has negative feelings;

+ hiding inside clothes to become invisible;

+ deteriorating attendance or punctuality;

+ deteriorating profile across areas of learning and development.

This is not an exhaustive list and specific mental health needs have specific warning signs. If you are concerned about a child, then you should discuss your concerns with the designated safeguarding lead or person with responsibility for special educational needs. You should also discuss your concerns with the parent. Some of these warning signs may need to be carefully considered. For example, hiding inside clothes can happen quite spontaneously and might not indicate that children have a mental health need. If this behaviour is prolonged then it might require further investigation. Soling can arise from a physical or medical problem and is common in children from birth to four years old. However, if it extends well beyond this then it might need further investigation.

CRITICAL QUESTIONS

+ What are the controversies relating to a diagnosis of mental ill-health in the early years?

+ What are the risks associated with labelling children?

+ How easy is it to gain a diagnosis of mental ill-health in infants?

It is important to remember that young children may display poor behaviour because they have underdeveloped self-regulation skills rather than poor mental health. If behaviours are short-term, this could indicate that self-regulation skills need further development. If the behaviour is exhibited over a long period of time, this could indicate that the child has a mental health need. It is important to observe the child in a range of contexts and to communicate your concerns with parents, other practitioners, health visitors and other external professionals.

In 2017:

🕐 5.5 per cent of pre-school children aged 2–4 years had at least one mental health disorder;

🕐 1.3 per cent of pre-school children aged 2–4 years had sleeping disorders;

🕐 boys aged 2–4 years were more likely to have mental ill-health than girls.

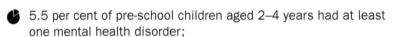

(https://files.digital.nhs.uk/F6/A5706C/MHCYP%202017%20Summary.pdf)

ANXIETY

Anxiety disorders range in both type and severity. Children with general anxiety disorder may demonstrate anxiety in a range of situations, while children with specific phobias usually experience anxiety in relation to very specific situations. Some young children may experience separation anxiety; this is anxiety resulting from separation from significant individuals in their lives. In addition, children who experience social phobias tend to experience anxiety in specific social situations. Children with anxiety may display a range of symptoms. These may include:

+ fearfulness, irritability, panic, breathlessness and sleep deprivation;

+ headaches;

+ stomach aches;

+ tearfulness;

+ sweating;

+ being clingy.

Your observations will help you to identify the factors that result in the child developing anxiety. You should set small, achievable goals for the child and praise them regularly when they achieve a goal. You should not feel afraid to talk to children about your own anxieties and how you overcame them. Children's stories that focus on the theme of anxiety are also a useful way of normalising anxiety because they help children to recognise that other people also experience anxiety.

CRITICAL QUESTIONS

+ What factors in the setting might result in a child becoming anxious? Explain your answer.

+ How can you reduce anxiety in the setting?

STRESS

Stress and anxiety are often used interchangeably but they are different things. A child may feel stressed but not anxious, although stress can sometimes result in the child developing anxiety or depression. Signs of stress include:

+ being irritable;

+ feeling over-burdened;

+ inability to relax;

+ lack of humour;

+ being aggressive;

+ being impatient or becoming wound-up.

Early childhood should not be a time when children experience stress. Children learn better when they are relaxed and free of pressure. Providing children with opportunities to learn in a rich, stimulating and enabling learning environment will reduce levels of stress. Learning through play and learning in the outdoors will also facilitate enjoyment in learning. Despite this, some children may demonstrate signs of stress and the factors that have resulted in this might be situated in the setting, family or community. Providing children with some simple strategies for managing stress will help children to control their stress.

CRITICAL QUESTIONS

+ What factors might result in a child becoming stressed? Explain your answer.

+ What strategies might you use that will help children to manage their stress? Explain your answer.

DEPRESSION

Depression falls along a spectrum from mild to severe. It can fluctuate depending on personal experiences and it can affect a child's learning and development across all aspects of the Early Years Foundation Stage framework. Children may start to distance themselves from others, become withdrawn, tearful, quiet and demonstrate low mood. Other common signs include:

+ displaying lack of interest in activities;

+ isolating themselves from others;

+ tiredness;

+ feeling hopeless or worthless.

The causes of childhood depression are multifaceted and complex. Family factors may be responsible for depression, particularly if children have experienced abuse, neglect, family conflict or parental separation.

Children may become depressed when they are separated from their parents during the day. However, there is a distinction between experiencing a low mood and being depressed. Depression affects participation in normal day-to-day activities, whereas people can experience a low mood and function relatively well. Your observations of the child in a range of contexts will indicate whether they have a low mood or are depressed. You can support them by assigning them to a key worker that they are most comfortable with. Establishing clear, consistent routines and engaging them in physical and social activities are also good strategies for addressing depression. Most importantly, you need to establish warm, positive and trusting relationships with children to show them that you care.

GRIEF AND LOSS

Children can experience grief through the death of a parent, sibling, other family member or friend. They might also experience grief following the death of a pet. Children might grieve for friendships they once had and now do not, especially if they have moved to a new setting, town, city or country. Children might feel a sense of loss if they have experienced permanent or temporary separation from their parents or other family members. They might also experience feelings of loss during times of transition, for example, when they move from home to pre-school. Grief and loss might result in anxiety, depression or even conduct disorders.

In relation to grief, practitioners should not be afraid to use the word 'death', even with younger children. You might say 'I was sorry to hear that your dog has died'. It is better to be honest with young children rather than trying to protect them from the truth. When children return to the setting following the death of someone close, it is important to establish a clear sense of routine.

You should not expect the child to grieve for a specific period. Some children need longer than others to grieve. Others will appear to be coping but they may still feel sad. It is often surprising how quickly young children appear to recover following the death of a loved one or a pet. They may not have fully comprehended the permanency of death and the grief might be delayed. This delay might extend over several years. Children's ability to cope with grief may be affected by the circumstances of the death, their own resilience and access to support networks.

Sometimes following a period of grief, a child may appear to be coping well but something very specific may trigger a memory or an emotion.

This might be a birthday, a special occasion, a place or even a happy event that they wish the deceased person could share. You will need to be patient with the child and reassure them that this is not something they should feel bad about. Providing children with the opportunity to hear and read stories that address grief is a useful way of educating them about grief. Stories that address grief and loss through pets are particularly useful for very young children. Some children may respond well to having 'quiet time' in a space where they can reflect upon their feelings. You should not be afraid to talk to children about your own experiences of grief.

CASE STUDY

Alex was three years old. His mother was diagnosed with terminal cancer a year ago and had recently died. Prior to the death, Alex's parents prepared him by explaining what was going to happen. They created a photograph album of special family memories for Alex to keep after the death. When Alex returned to pre-school he was allowed to take the album into the setting. If he felt sad he was allowed to spend time looking at the photographs of his family. On his first day back in the setting, his key worker, Helen, talked to Alex about the death of his mother. Helen explained to Alex that she was sorry to hear about his mother's death and she spent some time with him looking at the photographs. It was not long before Alex wanted to join in with all of the activities in the setting. He loved going in the writing area and he chose to draw a picture of his mother and write a simple message to her. For several weeks Helen monitored Alex closely to check on his mood. If she noticed that he appeared to be sad, withdrawn, tearful or lonely then she spent some time with him. Helen kept in regular contact with Alex's father for several weeks and together they agreed on how to support Alex both at home and in the setting.

SELF-HARM

Signs of self-harm include:

+ self-cutting;

+ burning;

+ scratching;

+ biting;

+ hair pulling;

+ head banging.

The reasons for self-harm are complex and multifaceted but it is not usually correct to assume that a child will self-harm to gain attention. They might self-harm to divert an emotional pain into a physical pain but rarely do they self-harm to gain attention. Self-harm can also be a form of self-punishment if children think that something is their fault.

If you notice or suspect that a child is self-harming, it is important to suspend negative judgement. Your role is to try to understand the child and find ways of helping them. You should demonstrate empathy. You also discuss your concerns with relevant people in the setting to agree on the most appropriate response.

ATTACHMENT DISORDERS

The work of Bowlby helped to demonstrate the significance of positive attachments between children and their primary caregivers. In cases where loving, caring and secure attachments are not formed because of the family context, this can have a detrimental impact on the child's sense of self and their behaviour. These children may be withdrawn, demonstrate anti-social behaviour, have low confidence and a negative perception of their abilities. This is not an exhaustive list, but it does demonstrate the range of traits that might be demonstrated.

It is critical that you focus on developing relationships that are consistently positive so that the child can start to trust you and feel safe. The use of praise, encouragement and rewards will support the development of a healthy relationship between the child and the adult. Some children may require specific intervention to support them with the development of their social and emotional skills. Others may require self-esteem enhancing interventions to build a positive sense of self.

CONDUCT DISORDERS

Some children demonstrate poor behaviour as they learn to adapt to the behavioural expectations in the setting. Through the support of practitioners, most children learn to adjust their behaviour. Conduct disorders are severe and persistent patterns of negative behaviour.

Identifying these early will enable you to provide support to help the child to improve their behaviour. Signs of conduct disorders include:

+ *being argumentative, angry, uncooperative or irritable;*

+ *having frequent tantrums and angry outbursts;*

+ *being aggressive;*

+ *being constantly defiant;*

+ *blaming others for things that go wrong;*

+ *telling lies regularly;*

+ *appearing cruel and lacking empathy for other children;*

+ *seeking out risky experiences without thinking about the consequences.*

(www.mentallyhealthyschools.org.uk/mental-health-needs/
challenging-behaviours)

You can support children with conduct disorders by providing them with an individual rewards system through which positive behaviour is acknowledged and celebrated. You should involve the child and their parent(s) in establishing behaviour goals and in reviewing progress. Some children might need a curriculum that explicitly teaches them social and emotional skills. Often poor behaviour is an attempt by the child to communicate a need. Most children with challenging behaviour can be supported to change their behaviour patterns and they can learn to adjust their behaviour in different contexts with the right support. You might want to consider keeping a behaviour diary, which will enable you to identify possible triggers for behaviour. Teaching children the skills of conflict resolution is also effective and gives the child some owner-ship. Demonstrating unconditional positive regard for the child is vital, regardless of their behaviour.

CRITICAL QUESTIONS

+ What individual factors may result in conduct disorders?
  Explain your answer.

+ What family-related factors may result in conduct disorders?
  Explain your answer.

+ What factors in the setting may result in conduct disorders?
  Explain your answer.

CASE STUDY

Tom was aged five and demonstrated signs of conduct disorder. He was frequently defiant to practitioners. He regularly refused to complete tasks and he had started to become physically aggressive towards other children. Tom was exposed to parental conflict in the home and his mother was a victim of domestic violence. Tom's father was the perpetrator of the violence. Sarah, his key worker, was aware of the situation in Tom's home and the case had already been referred to social care services.

Sarah focused on noticing when Tom demonstrated positive behaviour. All positive behaviour was rewarded using an individual rewards system that was designed for Tom. Tom was given five opportunities to gain rewards during the day: at the end of each of the two morning sessions, the end of the afternoon session, during lunch time and during the morning break. Stamps were attached to a daily reward chart for positive behaviour and Tom was given a reward at the end of the day if he had gained three out of the five possible stamps.

In 2017:

- 2.5 per cent of pre-school children aged 2–4 years had a behavioural disorder;

- 1.9 per cent of pre-school children aged 2–4 years had oppositional defiant disorder.

(https://files.digital.nhs.uk/F6/A5706C/
MHCYP%202017%20Summary.pdf)

There is a widespread perception that children and young people today experience greater mental ill-health than previous generations (Murphy and Fonagy, 2013).

However, increases in diagnoses do not necessarily mean that mental illness is increasing, because increases can be affected by changes in awareness, knowledge, stigma and understanding of what constitutes mental disorder (Rüsch et al, 2012).

SUMMARY

This chapter has identified the common types of mental ill-health in early childhood. It has provided useful strategies that you can use to support children with specific needs. The range of factors affecting children's mental health have also been explained and examples have been identified and discussed. The chapter provides some key warning signs of mental ill-health and explains what practitioners may notice during their observations of children in different contexts.

CHECKLIST

This chapter has addressed:

✓ the common types of mental ill-health experienced during early childhood;

✓ the factors affecting children's mental ill-health;

✓ the actions and strategies that practitioners can use to identify and support children's needs;

✓ key warning signs that indicate potential mental ill-health in children.

FURTHER READING

Vohra, S (2018) *Mental Health in Children and Young People: Spotting Symptoms and Seeking Help Early*. London: Sheldon Press.

✛ CHAPTER 7

THE ROLE OF HIGH-QUALITY PROVISION IN THE EARLY YEARS IN MITIGATING RISK

PROFESSIONAL LINKS

This chapter addresses the following:

⬡ *Bold Beginnings: The Reception Curriculum in a Sample of Good and Outstanding Primary Schools* (Ofsted, 2017).

CHAPTER OBJECTIVES

By the end of this chapter you will understand:

+ the importance of play-based learning in the early years;

+ indicators of quality provision in the early years;

+ the relationship between quality provision and children's well-being.

INTRODUCTION

Research on high-quality early years provision emphasises the important role that learning through play makes to children's learning and development. This is reflected in the Early Years Foundation Stage framework and the associated characteristics of effective learning. Learning through play provides a natural way for young children to learn. It supports their physical, social, emotional and intellectual development and it supports the development of positive well-being. However, perspectives on learning in the early years are not shared between individuals, within and across groups with different vested interests. The *Bold Beginnings* (Ofsted, 2017) report that is addressed in this chapter has been controversial in England because it marks a departure from the principles of effective learning in the EYFS framework through its emphasis on the direct teaching of literacy and mathematics in the Reception year. Academics, early years organisations and practitioners have responded to the recommendations with emotion, anger and evidence-based critiques to emphasise the critical importance of play-based learning in the early years and the detrimental effects of introducing formal teaching too early. However, it is questionable whether one framework spanning birth to five years can meet the needs of all children and it is a matter of debate about whether the role of the Reception year is to prepare children for the challenges of the national curriculum or whether it should be treated as a distinct phase of children's education. This chapter will address the elements of effective pedagogy in the early years and it will consider the implications of transitions for children's mental health and well-being.

PROMOTING LEARNING IN THE EARLY YEARS

Effective pedagogy in the early years involves understanding of how children learn and develop (Stewart and Pugh, 2007) so that subsequent learning builds on what children already know and can do. In the early years, particular emphasis should be given to supporting children's physical, social, emotional, language and communication development (Heckman, 2006; Goswami, 2015; Tickell, 2011). These aspects of development make positive contributions to the learning of specific areas of learning such as reading, writing and mathematics (Goddard-Blythe, 2017).

In addition, play and playfulness in learning help to promote the dispositions and skills to underpin that learning, such as self-regulation (Broadhead et al, 2010; Moyles, 2015; Rogers, 2011; Whitebread and Bingham, 2014). Research suggests that developing children's self-regulation skills and executive functions supports subsequent learning and development beyond the early years (Whitebread and Bingham, 2014; Diamond et al, 2007; Diamond, 2013) and more recent evidence indicates that the development of executive functions is strongly indicative of school success (Kangas et al, 2015). Diamond's research (2013) suggests that a range of executive functions are needed to support children's learning and development. The research suggests that these aspects of development are more important than intelligence or children's abilities in reading or mathematics (Blair and Diamond, 2008). Three core executive functions are suggested which appear to be associated with long-term attainment and which are vital for children's development. These are:

+ cognitive flexibility: the ability to switch perspectives;

+ inhibitory control: the ability to stay focused on a specific task despite distraction;

+ working memory: the ability to hold information in mind and mentally work with it, the ability to link concepts and ideas and process multiple instructions in sequence.

Snowling et al (2011) found a relationship between language and communication and later attainment. They presented considerable evidence to show that language skills are among the best predictors of educational success. This provides a clear rationale for play-based learning. Through immersing children in a rich language environment, children develop key skills that are essential for subsequent development in reading and writing. Through play they develop and use vocabulary and start to use language for communication. These skills underpin literacy development. In addition, Grissmer et al (2010) found that motor skills in early childhood were significant predictors of achievement in literacy and mathematics following the early years phase of education. Well-planned play-based learning provides children with valuable opportunities to develop their gross and fine motor skills and this supports subsequent development in writing. Through play children develop their social skills. They learn the skills of social interaction, social communication, turn-taking, sharing, problem-solving and conflict resolution. Through pretend play and role-play, they also develop their imagination skills which are critical for creativity and literacy development. Social skills have been found to be important predictors of positive mental health and well-being (Goodman et al, 2015).

CRITICAL QUESTIONS

+ What are the tensions associated with learning through play in the Reception year?

+ How can the most able children be challenged through play in the early years?

+ What is the role of play-based learning in supporting children's learning and development?

+ What are the advantages of adult interactions in children's play and are there any associated limitations?

MANAGING TRANSITIONS TO PRE-SCHOOL AND NURSERY

While some children are ready to make the transition from home to pre-school, for others this can be a difficult time that causes significant stress and anxiety. While most children adapt quickly to this transition, for others the process of adaption takes longer, and these children will require greater support. The role of the key worker is critical in facilitating a smooth transition. The key worker should establish positive, warm and trusting relationships with the children in their care so that children can quickly start to adapt to the setting. It is crucial to ensure that there is regular communication between parents and practitioners so that any concerns about the child can be quickly addressed. Providing children with an enabling learning environment that is challenging, stimulating and interesting will help children to adapt to the setting quickly. Developing clear, consistent routines in the setting will provide children with a sense of security. Supporting children to develop friendships is critical to ensuring that they experience a sense of belonging in the setting and developing a culture of inclusion, in which children are valued, respected and happy will support them in adapting to the setting. Visits to the setting prior to them transitioning will provide them with opportunities to meet the practitioners, to become familiar with the environment and to meet new friends. This is an effective strategy for facilitating a smooth transition.

MANAGING TRANSITIONS TO RECEPTION

In 2017 Ofsted published a report titled *Bold Beginnings: The Reception Curriculum in a Sample of Good and Outstanding Primary Schools*. The report made several claims about high-quality practice in the Reception year. These are outlined below.

In effective settings:

+ reading was at the heart of the curriculum;

+ systematic synthetic phonics played a critical role in teaching children the alphabetic code;

+ good phonics teaching supported children's early writing;

+ practical equipment to support children's grasp of numbers was used and more formal, written recording was introduced, but only when children's understanding was secure and automatic;

+ checks of children's phonics knowledge, standardised tests for reading and analysis of children's work provided the essential information that Year 1 teachers needed at the point of transition;

+ effective settings made sure that they gave reading, writing and mathematics enough direct teaching time every day.

Key recommendations in this report included the following:

+ *the teaching of reading, including systematic synthetic phonics, must be the core purpose of the Reception Year;*

+ *greater importance must be given to the teaching of numbers in building children's fluency in counting, recognising small numbers of items, comparing numbers and solving problems;*

+ *children should be taught correct pencil grip and how to sit correctly at a table;*

+ *enough time must be allocated each day to the direct teaching of reading, writing and mathematics, including frequent opportunities for children to practise and consolidate their skills.*

(Ofsted, 2017)

CRITICAL QUESTIONS

+ What are your views on these recommendations?

+ Why do you think Ofsted may have made these recommendations?

+ How might these recommendations impact on children's well-being and mental health?

The key points in the *Bold Beginnings* report emphasise the importance of the direct teaching of skills in literacy and mathematics, and this marks a move away from the play-based pedagogy advocated in the Early Years Foundation Stage framework. The report makes it clear that the focus on the direct teaching of reading, writing and mathematics in the Reception year will give children the best chance of being ready for the national curriculum. While some children may be ready for a more structured pedagogy in the Reception year, those who are working below the expectations of the Early Learning Goals may not be developmentally ready for narrower focus on literacy and mathematics; practitioners may need to focus on developing their social and emotional skills and therefore a play-based approach may be more appropriate. The *Bold Beginnings* report marks a move that signals the 'schoolification' of the early years. This is a dangerous move because it can result in a curriculum that is not developmentally appropriate for children and this could have a significant detrimental effect on their mental health.

According to the *Bold Beginnings* report:

A child's early education lasts a lifetime. Done well, it can mean the difference between gaining seven Bs at GCSE compared with seven Cs.

(Ofsted, 2017)

The EPPE study identified effective pedagogic approaches and highlighted that more *'sustained shared thinking'* (Sylva et al, 2004, p 1) was observed in settings where children made the most progress. Sustained shared thinking occurs when two or more individuals work together to solve a problem, clarify a concept, evaluate an activity or extend a narrative. Skilled practitioners can develop children's thinking in relation to a problem, concept or task using open-ended questioning to move children through their zone of proximal development. The study found that in effective settings adults modelled skills and often combined modelling with sustained periods of shared thinking: open-ended questioning and modelling were also associated with better cognitive achievement (Sylva et al, 2004).

CASE STUDY

Hedgehog Primary School was recently inspected and graded inadequate across all areas of the inspection framework. The inspectors highlighted in their report that children in the Reception class were working below the expected level of attainment specified in the Early Learning Goals. The school was situated in an area of social deprivation and children entered the Reception class with very low skills in communication and language. Many children, upon entry, were unable to regulate their feelings and found it difficult to adhere to rules. By March the children had made significant progress from their baseline entry levels, but their attainment was low. Josh, the Reception teacher, had focused on developing a rich, stimulating and enabling play-based learning environment that supported children's progress across all areas of learning and development.

Following the inspection, the head teacher asked to meet with Josh to discuss the inspection findings. Josh was instructed to remove all areas in the classroom that enabled children to initiate their own play. Josh was told to create a seating plan and to seat the children in a fixed place with tables arranged in pairs. The head teacher asked Josh to create timetabled reading, writing and mathematics lessons every morning and the afternoon sessions were to be used for providing same-day interventions for those children who had developed misconceptions during the morning lessons. Josh was not happy with the new arrangements, but he felt that he had no choice but to comply with the expectations of his head teacher.

CRITICAL QUESTIONS

+ What are your views in relation to the decisions that were made in this meeting?

+ Had you been Josh, how might you have responded to the head teacher?

According to the *Bold Beginnings* report:

- In 2016, around one third of Reception-aged children did not have the essential knowledge and understanding they needed to reach a good level of development by the age of five.

- The outcomes for disadvantaged children were far worse. Only just over half had the knowledge and understanding needed to secure a positive start to Year 1.

- In 2016–17, the quality of early years provision was inadequate in 84 schools and required improvement in a further 331 of those inspected that year.

(Ofsted, 2017)

In the EPPE study, the balance of who initiated the activities, staff or child, was about equal in the most effective settings. Similarly, in effective settings the extent to which staff members extended child-initiated interactions was important. The research found that almost half the child-initiated episodes that contained intellectual challenge included interventions from a staff member to extend the child's thinking. Also, freely chosen play activities often provided the best opportunities for adults to extend the child's thinking. The research suggested that extending the child-initiated play, coupled with the provision of adult-led group work, are the most effective vehicles to promote learning and development. Children's cognitive outcomes appeared to be directly related to the quantity and quality of the teacher/adult-planned and initiated focused group work.

The EPPE study found that the way in which behaviour is managed is critical to the quality of the provision; in effective settings practitioners encouraged children to resolve their own conflicts. In settings that were less effective there was often no follow-up on children's misbehaviour and, on many occasions, children were distracted or simply told to stop behaving inappropriately.

(Sylva et al, 2004)

CASE STUDY

In a pre-school setting in the north of England the practitioners noticed that several children were displaying signs of conduct disorders. They found it difficult to follow rules and routines and they were frequently defiant to the requests of the practitioners. They were often physically aggressive to other children in the setting and sometimes they were physically aggressive to practitioners. The key workers who were responsible for these children each met with the parents, only to be informed by the parents that they did not experience these problems at home. The parents blamed the practitioners for the problems rather than being honest about their own experiences of managing their behaviour.

The practitioners introduced a social and emotional curriculum. The children who demonstrated signs of conduct behaviour received daily intervention to support them in developing their social skills and their understanding of feelings using stories and puppets. In addition, the sessions focused on enhancing the children's feelings of self-worth;

in one session the children were supported to help them understand the things that they were good at. They were helped to understand that in some contexts they were already demonstrating the skills that they needed to demonstrate in the setting. For example, four of the children had pets so the practitioner supported them to understand that they could already demonstrate that they were caring and able to follow rules because they demonstrated these skills when they looked after their pets. They were supported to understand that they simply needed to do the same things in the setting. One session focused on how they cared for other members of their family. It was clear that the children already had the skills of being able to care and demonstrate kindness and respect towards others, so the practitioner supported them to understand that they needed to transfer these skills into the setting.

Finally, the key workers developed an individual reward system which was bespoke to each child. Children received regular rewards for good behaviour and the practitioners focused on noticing times when good behaviour was demonstrated. Each child was also provided with a visual timetable so that they could identify the sequence of activities that had to be completed during each day. These children initially needed a more structured approach to learning, and therefore free-flow play was not appropriate for them until they were able to regulate their emotions. They were required to complete specific tasks in a specific order. One of the activities on the visual timetable included a task that related to the child's interests. If they refused to complete a task, they were reminded about the sequence of activities on the visual timetable and informed that if they refused to complete a task, this would result in them not progressing through the sequence and therefore they would be unable to complete the task that related to their own interests.

To facilitate positive relationships with the parents, the practitioners completed a daily diary that only recorded positive behaviours the child had demonstrated that day. Messages were written to parents to communicate positive behaviours and parents were encouraged to document positive behaviours noticed at home to bring these to the attention of the practitioners.

SUMMARY

This chapter has emphasised the importance of learning through play on a child's development in the early years. The benefits of learning through play have been identified and the chapter has linked these to children's physical, social, emotional and intellectual development and thus positive well-being. It has also considered the elements of effective pedagogy in the early years and the implications of transition for children's mental health and well-being.

CHECKLIST

This chapter has addressed:

✓ the role of play-based learning and its impact on children's development;

✓ the common indicators of high-quality and effective provision in the early years;

✓ the importance of high-quality and effective provision and its impact on children's well-being.

FURTHER READING

Bottrill, G (2018) *Can I Go and Play Now? Rethinking the Early Years*. London: Sage.

The Key for School Leaders. [online] Available at: https:// schoolleaders.thekeysupport.com (accessed 28 February 2019).

PACEY: Professional Association for Childcare and Early Years. [online] Available at: www.pacey.org.uk/working-in-childcare/spotlight-on/ creating-enabling-environments (accessed 28 February 2019).

Pre-School Learning Alliance. [online] Available at: www.pre-school.org. uk/enabling-environments (accessed 28 February 2019).

✚ CHAPTER 8

MENTAL HEALTH IN THE EARLY YEARS FOUNDATION STAGE FRAMEWORK

PROFESSIONAL LINKS

This chapter addresses the following:

Department for Education (2017) *Statutory Framework for the Early Years Foundation Stage: Setting the Standards for Learning, Development and Care for Children from Birth to Five*. London: DfE.

CHAPTER OBJECTIVES

By the end of this chapter you will understand:

+ how the principles of the early years framework support children to be mentally healthy;

+ the role of the areas of learning and development in supporting children's mental health;

+ the role of the key person;

+ the principles that underpin assessment and their role in supporting children to be mentally healthy.

INTRODUCTION

This chapter addresses how aspects of the Early Years Foundation Stage framework can support children to be mentally healthy. While the most significant link to mental health in the framework is through personal, social and emotional development, you will learn about how other aspects of the framework can support children's mental health. Specifically, this chapter addresses the principles of the EYFS and their contribution to children's mental health. It also covers the areas of learning and their role in supporting positive well-being. The chapter also examines the role of assessment in supporting children's mental health in the context of attentive adults observing children, understanding individual children's needs and supporting their learning and development. Finally, the contribution of the characteristics of effective teaching and learning to children's confidence and self-worth are examined.

THE PRINCIPLES OF THE FRAMEWORK

Four principles shape practice in early years settings. These are summarised below:

+ *every child is a unique child, who is constantly learning and can be resilient, capable, confident and self-assured;*

+ *children learn to be strong and independent through positive relationships;*

+ *children learn and develop well in enabling environments, in which their experiences respond to their individual needs and there is a strong partnership between practitioners and parents and/or carers;*

+ *children develop and learn in different ways.*

(DfE, 2017)

CRITICAL QUESTIONS

+ How do you address these principles in your setting?

+ How might you further embed these principles?

If these principles are addressed, they will support children to be mentally healthy. Valuing each child as a unique learner will help children to develop a positive sense of identity and culture. The framework emphasises that you should respect and value all children and families and by doing this you will support children to develop a positive sense of self-worth. This is critical for supporting children to be mentally healthy. You should establish warm, loving and positive relationships with children to support them in feeling included in the setting and experiencing a sense of belonging. You should value all achievements, however small, recognising that small steps in learning and development can constitute significant milestones for children. Valuing all achievements will promote self-worth, confidence and motivation. Good practice in the early years supports children in learning, offers opportunities to extend learning and encourages children to develop resilience when faced with challenging tasks. This support a child's well-being, rather than their becoming anxious and concerned about possible failure. The environment enables a safe exploration of new experiences. You should encourage children to persevere with tasks that they find challenging and celebrate their achievements once they have mastered a new skill. Children should be given opportunities to learn through playful experiences. Through well-planned play, developed from your observations of children's interests and their current stage of development, children will be stimulated and operating at their highest level of development (Vygotsky, 1978). Your role as a practitioner is to plan opportunities for child-initiated playful learning that build on children's existing capabilities. Activities and learning opportunities should ideally grow organically from the children's needs and interests.

THE PRIME AREAS OF LEARNING

The prime areas of learning underpin the specific areas and for this reason it is important that greater emphasis is placed on the prime areas, particularly in the 0–3 age range. Supporting the development of children's skills in these areas will help to develop their confidence and facilitate a positive feeling of self-worth, which is essential for good mental health.

COMMUNICATION AND LANGUAGE

Developing children's language skills is essential for subsequent development in reading and writing. Some children do not have well developed communication skills. They may not talk so much, but this is where the experienced practitioner has an important role to play, offering support to join in talk, to extend vocabulary and confidence. This age group benefits from songs, nursery rhymes, short stories, playing with puppets and listening to others in conversation. This may not be a planned activity but it is integral to good practice and should take place throughout the setting. Initially very young children will communicate through glances and responding to touch and noise; as they grow they begin to turn their head to a voice or sound. Babies learn to make noises to get someone's attention. The attentive carer recognises what the different cries mean. As the baby grows it engages in communication exchange by using eye-contact and gesture. Even after they have developed language skills, some children will be reluctant to speak and express themselves verbally. You can support them by encouraging them to use other forms of expression such as mark-making, drawing, making choices from pictures, pointing and gesture. Through adopting a sensitive and patient approach, you can support children to learn to express themselves verbally and children who are non-verbal can be supported to express themselves through using signs and symbols, including Makaton. Once children have the confidence to express themselves, they can be supported to talk about how they feel if they are exhibiting low mood, anger or upset. If they are not confident in talking to you about their feelings, you can encourage them to talk to puppets. Talking about how they feel or expressing their feelings through non-verbal communication is an important tool to support them in being mentally healthy. If they feel sad, frightened, worried or angry, it is important that they are able to express these feelings. Expressing their feelings to others is a help-seeking strategy that can prevent problems from escalating.

PHYSICAL DEVELOPMENT

Supporting children's physical development in the early years is critical because research has identified a correlation between physical activity and mental health. Biddle and Asare's (2011) review combines much of this research and evidences the positive correlation between physical activity and positive mental health while also demonstrating the link between sedentary screen-time and mental ill-health. However, physical development in the early years is wider than physical activity. It includes the development of gross and fine motor skills, and fine motor skills development in particular underpins children's development in writing. Proficiency in fine motor skills will give children the confidence to hold and control a pencil, which is a critical aspect of their subsequent development. Using a pencil correctly is a learned skill built up gradually over time. It starts with picking up smaller and smaller objects using the fingers. Playing with objects such as bricks will also support the development of motor skills. You can gradually develop more complex manipulation skills using smaller objects, which builds the fine motor muscles. Finger painting, printing and painting using large fat brushes all underpin the development of motor skills, which supports subsequent development in writing. These developmentally appropriate activities lead to success and build confidence. Once children master the skills of making marks and feel comfortable using different marks then they are more likely to experiment and develop drawing skills. This is only possible when children feel confident and safe trying something new. Asking them to control a pencil, write or draw before they are developmentally ready to do so can result in anxiety, reduced confidence and poor self-worth. If you notice that a child is struggling to control a pencil they might require a fine motor skills intervention rather than a writing intervention. Understanding how children learn and develop will enable you to tailor the interventions to the needs of the child, thus ensuring that interventions are developmentally appropriate. This will build confidence and self-esteem.

PERSONAL, SOCIAL AND EMOTIONAL DEVELOPMENT

Personal social and emotional development is a significant aspect that underpins their mental health. It includes:

+ self-confidence and self-awareness;

+ managing feelings and behaviour;

+ making relationships.

As a practitioner you play a critical role in developing children's self-confidence. This helps them to develop positive self-worth and supports them to take risks in their learning. Confidence and self-worth help children to develop a positive view of themselves and this supports them in being mentally healthy. Supporting children to express and regulate their feelings will also help them to develop a positive view of themselves. Children's behaviour is usually an attempt to communicate an unmet need rather than a sign of deliberate defiance. Your role as a practitioner is to help children to communicate their needs in positive ways rather than through negative behaviours. This will support them in developing a positive self-concept. Providing children with a social and emotional programme that explicitly focuses on feelings and the rules of social interaction will help them to adjust their behaviours in the context of the setting and develop empathy for others.

Establishing positive relationships is critical for well-being. Human beings are wired for social connectivity, unless they have specific needs such as autism, and social interactions help children to feel included, experience a sense of belonging and stay mentally healthy. Research has demonstrated the importance of social connectedness for positive mental health (Saeri et al, 2017) and the impact of social isolation on children's mental ill-health (Matthews et al, 2015).

CASE STUDY

Aghala had recently experienced a mid-year transition and Aghala's new practitioner, Adrian, was concerned about her reluctance to speak and express herself verbally. Aghala's old practitioner, Abra, has confirmed that there were no concerns about Aghala throughout her time in her previous setting.

Adrian planned an activity to allow Aghala to summarise her feelings through drawing and then discuss these with another child. Aghala responded to this well and completed both activities. Adrian continued to repeat this activity on a weekly basis. For ten weeks, Aghala would not discuss her feelings with Adrian but she would communicate these to other children. Eventually, after ten weeks, Aghala discussed her drawings and explained to Adrian why she had chosen to draw what she had. Adrian's sensitive and patient approach supported Aghala and developed her confidence. Giving Aghala these different options to express her feelings supported her social connectedness and, in doing so, promoted her positive mental health.

THE SPECIFIC AREAS OF LEARNING

LITERACY

In literacy children develop their skills in reading and writing and there is a strong emphasis on the role of systematic synthetic phonics in supporting children to be readers and writers. This chapter has already considered the role of motor skills in underpinning writing development. Reading development is underpinned by visual discrimination skills, visual memory and phonological awareness skills, including developing sensitivity to rhyme. If children are struggling to master the skills of phoneme blending and segmenting, you should assess their visual and phonological awareness skills before providing synthetic phonics inter-vention. Some children may require interventions in these aspects before their phonemic awareness can be developed. You should ensure that rich opportunities to develop reading and writing are integrated into areas of continuous provision and you should provide children with exposure to a rich range of language, stories, information books and poems. Children should also have regular opportunities to listen to stories. Providing developmentally appropriate interventions will provide children with the skills they need to be effective readers and writers, foster self-worth and confidence, all of which are crucial for good mental health.

MATHEMATICS

The importance of children learning mathematics through access to practical, concrete resources cannot be overstated. This will ensure that mathematical concepts become firmly embedded in the child's mind. You should also plan opportunities to develop mathematical understanding through play-based learning so that children can apply the skills they have learned in adult-directed learning.

UNDERSTANDING THE WORLD

Through this area of learning, children learn about the differences between themselves and others, and among families, communities and traditions. This supports them in developing empathy for others and in fostering a climate of inclusion. These aspects of learning support children in being mentally healthy.

EXPRESSIVE ARTS AND DESIGN

Children can express their feelings through the arts; for example, through drawing or painting they can communicate how they feel. The arts provide a unique opportunity to learn through the senses. Through the arts children can develop their confidence, self-esteem and creativity. The arts as a whole play a critical role in supporting positive mental health.

THE CHARACTERISTICS OF EFFECTIVE TEACHING AND LEARNING

The characteristics of effective teaching and learning play a crucial role in supporting children's mental health. Consequently, you should integrate these characteristics into the planned and unplanned daily experiences of children. The characteristics are stated below:

+ *playing and exploring: children investigate and experience things, and 'have a go';*

+ *active learning: children concentrate and keep on trying if they encounter difficulties, and enjoy achievements;*

+ *creating and thinking critically: children have and develop their own ideas, make links between ideas, and develop strategies for doing things.*

(DfE, 2017)

Through supporting children to take risks in their learning and to persevere with activities that are either self-chosen or directed by an adult, children will experience a sense of achievement once they have mastered a task. This will develop confidence, self-worth and help them to understand that they can learn and develop through failure. You should ensure that children are never afraid to make mistakes in their learning. Through providing opportunities for playful active learning, children will be intrinsically motivated, engaged and obsessed in their learning. This supports them in being mentally healthy. Through celebrating their achievements with them you will develop their self-esteem. Through allowing to make their own decisions about their learning you will provide them with agency, which will breed confidence, motivation and positive mental health.

CRITICAL QUESTIONS

+ How do you address the characteristics for teaching and learning in your setting?

+ How might this be further enhanced?

OTHER IMPORTANT ASPECTS OF THE FRAMEWORK

Other key aspects of the Early Years Foundation Stage framework contribute to children's mental health. The framework states that:

Practitioners must consider the individual needs, interests, and stage of development of each child in their care and must use this information to plan a challenging and enjoyable experience for each child in all of the areas of learning and development.

(DfE, 2017, para 1.6)

CRITICAL QUESTIONS

+ How do you plan to address children's interests in your setting?

+ How might this aspect be further enhanced?

By planning developmentally appropriate learning opportunities children will experience success in their learning. You should take time to get to know the child, ascertain their strengths, areas for development and interests. You should aim to integrate their interests into the learning opportunities that you plan for them and planned activities should build on what children already know and can do. For children whose first language is not English, you should support them in using their home language within their play as well as using English. This cultural sensitivity will provide them with confidence and engender a sense of inclusion and belonging. These aspects underpin children's well-being. The framework states that:

For children whose home language is not English, providers must take reasonable steps to provide opportunities for children to develop and use their home language in play and learning, supporting their language development at home.

(DfE, 2017, para 1.7)

Planning opportunities to learn through a combination of child-initiated and adult-led learning will provide children with the best foundation for their learning. This mix of learning opportunities will help to develop their confidence. Children should be given opportunities to apply the skills, knowledge and understanding that you address through adult-led learning tasks in their child-initiated learning so that learning becomes embedded. The framework states that:

Each area of learning and development must be implemented through planned, purposeful play and through a mix of adult-led and child-initiated activity. Play is essential for children's development, building their confidence as they learn to explore, to think about problems, and relate to others. Children learn by leading their own play, and by taking part in play which is guided by adults.

(DfE, 2017, para 1.8)

Providing children with opportunities to self-initiate tasks will help to build children's confidence and provide them with ownership of their own learning.

KEY PERSON

The Early Years Foundation Stage framework states that '*Each child must be assigned a key person. Their role is to help ensure that every child's care is tailored to meet their individual needs*' (DfE, 2017, para 3.27). Your role as a key worker is to establish warm, positive and trusting relationships with children in your care. You should value their identities and families and you should help children to recognise that you believe in them. Your role in building children's confidence and empowering them to express their views and feelings cannot be overstated. For children who have no attachment figure at home, your role is critical in helping children to feel safe, secure, loved and valued.

SPECIAL EDUCATIONAL NEEDS

The Early Years Foundation Stage states that *'Providers must have arrangements in place to support children with SEN or disabilities'* (DfE, 2017, para 3.67). In the Code of Practice for Special Educational Needs and Disabilities (DfE and DoH, 2015), mental health is a recognised special educational need and/or disability. If you identify that a child has a mental health need, you should discuss this with the special educational needs and disability co-ordinator, the child's parent(s) or carer(s) and the child. If the child is identified as needing special educational needs support then practitioners are responsible for implementing a Graduated Approach to meet their needs. This is outlined below.

+ *Assess: assess the child's current need(s) to ascertain the starting points for planning;*

+ *Plan: plan intervention(s) to build on the child's existing capabilities;*

+ *Do: implement interventions to address the identified need(s);*

+ *Review: monitor the impact of the interventions to ascertain if they were successful.*

(DfE and DoH, 2015)

In the EPPE study (Sylva et al, 2004), research has explored the impact of pre-school on the impact of children with different kinds of needs. This research demonstrates that pre-school is particularly beneficial to those children who are disadvantaged. Of these children, the study found that one in three children were 'at risk' of developing learning difficulties at the start of pre-school, although this fell to one in five by the time they started school. This demonstrates that pre-school can be an effective intervention for the reduction of special educational needs (SEN).

Data for 2017 for children aged 2–4 years shows that 8.4 per cent of boys had a mental disorder compared to 3.9 per cent of girls.

(Health and Social Care Information Centre, 2018)

ASSESSMENT

Assessment in the early years is conducted via observations of children's learning in a range of contexts. This enables you to identify what children know and can do within the context of their natural learning environment. This ensures that assessment is not de-contextualised from the process of learning and it does not place children under stress. Formal tests and assessment tasks increase the risk of stress and anxiety and are not appropriate in the early years. It is also important that assessment does not become a 'tick box' exercise by writing copious observations of children, which simply constitute evidence that is stored in a file. The purpose of any assessment should be to promote learning. If assessment becomes a bureaucratic exercise then its true purpose can be lost. You should only aim to produce evidence that will help you to advance children's learning and development; this will protect your own mental health as a practitioner.

MANAGING BEHAVIOUR

Children may struggle to adapt their behaviour from that which is acceptable in the home to the expectations of the setting. Instead of focusing on negative behaviour, it is better to notice and acknowledge positive behaviour in order to increase the chances of children repeating it. It is more effective to respond to misbehaviour in a calm and controlled way. The reasons why children demonstrate inappropriate behaviour are complex and multifaceted. They may be rooted in the child's social environment, individual biology or factors arising from the setting. Demonstrating unconditional positive regard to children is essential. Some children will require a structured social and emotional intervention to support them in developing appropriate behaviours. An individual reward system, bespoke to the child, may be effective in some instances.

CASE STUDY

Jordan's parents and his practitioner have different expectations of his behaviour and as a result of this Jordan finds it hard to adapt his behaviour when moving between these settings. Jordan's practitioner, Dan, has consulted with Jordan's parents and conversation is ongoing.

In the meantime, Dan has introduced a system that notices and acknowledges examples of Jordan's positive behaviour and Dan has noticed that Jordan has started to repeat these behaviours. Dan does still respond to misbehaviours, although these have reduced since he began to focus on positive behaviours. Dan is trialling these ideas in his setting and is sharing these resources with Jordan's parents who have agreed to trial the idea in their home setting.

- 2017 data for children aged 2–4 years shows the prevalence of behavioural disorders for different ethnic groups: 3.3 per cent of those who were white had a behavioural disorder compared to 0.3 per cent of children from black and minority ethnic groups.

- Also, 2 per cent of boys had oppositional defiant disorder compared to 1.6 per cent of girls.

(Health and Social Care Information Centre, 2018)

In the EPPE study (Sylva et al, 2004), balance between areas of learning was examined and its impact on developmental domains was highlighted. The study demonstrates that settings that emphasise literacy, maths, science/environment and children's diversity promote better attainment outcomes for children in subsequent academic years, and especially in reading and mathematics. The study also found that settings that were strong on these aspects of learning also tended to be strong on the social and behavioural aspects too.

CRITICAL QUESTIONS

+ How might a focus on 'curriculum', reading, writing and mathematics in the early years affect children's mental health?

+ Do you agree with the findings of the EPPE research? Explain your answer.

UNDERSTANDING AND RESPONDING TO BEHAVIOUR

Children may struggle to adapt their behaviour from that which is acceptable in the home to the expectations of the setting. Instead of focusing on negative behaviour, it is better to notice and acknowledge positive behaviour in order to increase the chances of children repeating it. It is more effective to respond to misbehaviour in a calm and controlled way. The reasons why children demonstrate inappropriate behaviour are complex and multifaceted. They may be rooted in the child's social environment, individual biology or factors arising from the setting. Demonstrating unconditional positive regard to children is essential. Some children will require a structured social and emotional intervention to support them in developing appropriate behaviours. An individual reward system, bespoke to the child, may be effective in some instances.

SUMMARY

This chapter has explained how the Early Years Foundation Stage framework supports children and promotes their mental health. It has linked this to personal, social and emotional development among other aspects of the framework. The principles of the Early Years Foundation Stage have been addressed and the areas of learning and their role in supporting positive well-being have been addressed. The importance of considering assessment and its impact on children's mental health is also emphasised and the characteristics of effective teaching and learning are covered and linked to children's confidence and self-worth.

CHECKLIST

This chapter has addressed:

✓ the principles of the early years framework;

✓ how these principles support children's positive mental health;

✓ the role of the areas of learning and development and the impact of these on children's mental health;

✓ the principles of assessment and the role of these in supporting children's positive mental health.

FURTHER READING

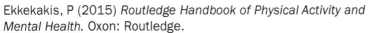

Ekkekakis, P (2015) *Routledge Handbook of Physical Activity and Mental Health.* Oxon: Routledge.

Williams, L (2016) *Positive Behaviour Management in Early Years Settings: An Essential Guide*. London: Jessica Kingsley Publishers.

✚ CONCLUSION

This book has provided an overview of some of the factors that may be associated with young children developing mental ill-health. It has outlined risk factors that may increase the likelihood of children developing mental ill-health and the protective factors that can mitigate against this. In addition, it has addressed common mental health needs that children may present with and explored themes such as attachment, resilience and self-regulation.

The importance of early positive attachments between children and their primary carer has been emphasised. Weak, unstable or non-existent attachments can lead to the development of social and emotional problems and the effects can extend into adult life. The importance of establishing warm, positive and trusting relationships with children has been emphasised throughout this book. In addition, the importance of treating children with respect, kindness and demonstrating empathy towards them has also been highlighted. The necessity to ensure that children feel included and experience a sense of belonging has also been discussed. Young children may experience stress and anxiety in relation to triggers that adults perceive as being relatively minor. However, this book has emphasised the importance of taking seriously children's concerns by acknowledging and affirming their feelings.

The book has argued that the 'schoolification' of early childhood is inappropriate. Introducing children to structured, adult-directed formal learning experiences too early is counterproductive to children's development and could have a detrimental impact on their mental health and well-being. Early years organisations, practitioners and academics are rightly concerned about the recommendations in the *Bold Beginnings* report, which appear not to have been informed by academic research, on how children learn and develop in the early years. There is a danger that an overemphasis on academic attainment in reading, writing and mathematics in the early years will result in the underdevelopment of children's personal, social and emotional skills. If these skills are not prioritised in the early years, this is likely to have a detrimental impact on their subsequent academic attainment and if children's exposure to language and communication is restricted in the early years this is likely to have a significant negative impact on their literacy development. Watering down the principles of the Early Years Foundation Stage, by introducing more structured learning, is likely to result in increases to mental ill-health in early childhood and a decline in academic attainment in the long-term.

➕ REFERENCES

Ainsworth, M D S, Blehar, M C, Waters, E and Wall, S (1978)
Patterns of Attachment: A Psychological Study of the Strange Situation.
New York, NY: Erlbaum.

Asbury, K and Plomin, R (2013)
*G is for Genes: The Impact of Genetics on Education and Achievement
(Understanding Children's Worlds).* Oxford: Wiley Blackwell.

Beck, U (1992)
Risk Society: Towards a New Modernity. London: Sage.

Biddle, S J H and Asare, M (2011)
Physical Activity and Mental Health in Children and Adolescents: A Review of
Reviews. *British Journal of Sports Medicine*, 45: 886–95.

Bingham, S and Whitebread, D (2012)
School Readiness: A Critical Review of Perspectives and Evidence. Croome
D'Abitot, Worcs: TACTYC-Association for the Professional Development of Early
Years Educators.

Blackburn, C (2010)
*Primary Framework: Teaching and Learning Strategies to Support Primary Aged
Students With Foetal Alcohol Spectrum Disorder (FASD).* London: National
Organisation for Foetal Alcohol Syndrome.

Blair, C (2002)
School Readiness: Integrating Cognition and Emotion in a Neurobiological
Conceptualization of Children's Functioning at School Entry. *American
Psychologist*, 57(2): 111–27.

Blair, C and Razza, A (2007)
Relating Effortful Control, Executive Function, and False Belief Understanding
to Emerging Math and Literacy Ability in Kindergarten. *Child Development*,
78(2): 647–63.

Blair, C and Diamond, A (2008)
Biological Processes in Prevention and Intervention: The Promotion of Self-
Regulation as a Means of Preventing School Failure. *Development and
Psychopathology*, 20(3): 899–911.

Blair, C and Raver, C C (2015)
School Readiness and Self-Regulation: A Developmental Psychobiological
Approach. *Annual Review of Psychology*, 66(1): 711–31.

Bodrova, E and Leong, D J (2007)
Tools of the Mind: The Vygotskian Approach to Early Childhood Education
(2nd edn). Columbus, OH: Merrill/Prentice Hall.

Bodrova, E and Leong, D J (2008)
Developing Self-Regulation in Kindergarten: Can We Keep All the Crickets in
the Basket? *Young Children*, 63: 56–8.

Bodrova, E and Leong, D J (2015)
Vygotskian and Post-Vygotskian Views on Children's Play. *American Journal of
Play*, 7(3): 371–88.

Bonnet, A and Bernard, M (2012)
The Learning of Resilience. *Education Horizons*, 12(2): 22–3.

Bowlby, J (1939)
Substitute Homes. *Mother and Child*, 3–7 April.

Bowlby, J (1940)
Psychological Aspects. In Padley, R and Cole, M (eds) *Evacuation
Survey: A Report to the Fabian Society*, pp 186–96. London: George
Routledge & Sons.

Bowlby, J (1952)
Maternal Care and Mental Health. Geneva, Switzerland: World Health
Organization.

Bowlby, J (1960)
Grief and Mourning in Infancy and Early Childhood. *The Psychoanalytic
Study of the Child*, 15: 9–52.

Bowlby, J (2012)
A Secure Base. Oxon: Routledge.

Bridges, L and Grolnick, W (1995)
The Development of Emotional Self-Regulation in Infancy and Early Childhood.
In Eisnberg, N (ed) *Social Development* (pp 185–211). New York, NY: Sage.

Broadhead, P, Howard, J and Wood, E (2010)
Play and Learning in the Early Years: From Research to Practice.
London: Sage.

Bronfenbrenner, U (1979)
The Ecology of Human Development: Experiments by Nature and Design. Cambridge, MA: Harvard University Press.

Bronfenbrenner, U (2005)
The Developing Ecology of Human Development: Paradigm Lost or Paradigm Regained. In Bronfenbrenner, U (ed) Making Human Beings Human: Bioecological Perspectives on Human Development. Thousand Oaks, CA: Sage.

Brookman-Frazee, L, Drahota, A, Stadnick, N and Palinkas, L A (2012)
Therapist Perspectives on Community Mental Health Services for Children with Autism Spectrum Disorders. Administration and Policy in Mental Health and Mental Health Services Research, 39(5): 365–73.

Brookman-Frazee, L, Stadnick, N, Chlebowski, C, Baker-Ericzén, M and Ganger, W (2018)
Characterizing Psychiatric Comorbidity in Children with Autism Spectrum Disorder Receiving Publicly Funded Mental Health Services. Autism, 22(8): 938–52.

Calear, A L and Christensen, H (2010)
Systematic Review of School-Based Prevention and Early Intervention Programs for Depression. Journal of Adolescence, 33(3): 429–38.

Catterick, M and Curran, L (2014)
Understanding Fetal Alcohol Spectrum Disorder: A Guide to FASD for Parents, Carers and Professionals. London: Jessica Kingsley Publishers.

Center on the Developing Child at Harvard University (2014)
Enhancing and Practicing Executive Function Skills with Children from Infancy to Adolescence. [online] Available at: www.developingchild.harvard.edu (accessed 28 February 2019).

Department for Education (DfE) (2015)
Mental Health and Behaviour in Schools: Departmental Advice for School Staff. London: DfE.

Department for Education (DfE) (2017)
Statutory Framework for the Early Years Foundation Stage: Setting the Standards for Learning, Development and Care for Children from Birth to Five. London: DfE.

Department for Education (DfE) (2018)
International Early Learning and Child Well-Being Study (IELS) in England: Introduction to the Research. [online] Available at: www.gov.uk/government/publications (accessed 28 February 2019).

Department for Education and Department of Health (2015)
Special Educational Needs and Disability Code of Practice: 0 to 25 Years: Statutory Guidance for Organisations Which Work With and Support Children and Young People Who Have Special Educational Needs or Disabilities. London: DfE and DoH.

Diamond, A (2013)
Executive Functions. *Annual Review of Psychology*, 64: 135–68.

Diamond, A, Barnett, W S, Thomas, J and Munro, S (2007)
Preschool Program Improves Cognitive Control. *Science*, 3(18): 1387–8.

Dobia, B, Bodkin-Andrees, G, Parada, R, O'Rourke, V, Gilbert, S, Daley, A and Roffey, S (2014)
Aboriginal Girls Circle: Enhancing Connectedness and Promoting Resilience for Aboriginal Girls. Final Pilot Report. Sydney: University of Western Sydney.

Doll, B (2013)
Enhancing resilience in classrooms. In Goldstein, S and Brooks, R B (eds) *Handbook of Resiliency in Children* (pp 399–409). Dordrecht: Springer.

Dowling, E and Elliott, D (2012)
Understanding Children's Needs When Parents Separate. London: Speechmark Books.

Durlak, J E, Dymnicki, A B, Taylor, R D, Weissberg, R P and Schellinger, K B (2011)
The Impact of Enhancing Students Social and Emotional Learning: A Meta-Analysis of School-Based Universal Interventions. *Child Development*, 82(1): 405–32.

Early Intervention Foundation (2017)
EIF Policy Briefing: Social and Emotional Learning: Supporting Children and Young People's Mental Health. [online] Available at: www.eif.org.uk/files/pdf/social-emotional-learning-briefing.pdf (accessed 28 February 2019).

Education Policy Institute (2018)
Written evidence from the Education Policy Institute. [online] Available at: http://data.parliament.uk/writtenevidence/committeeevidence.svc/evidencedocument/health-and-social-care-committee/transforming-children-and-young-peoples-mental-health-provision/written/76777.pdf (accessed 28 February 2019).

Emerson, E and Hatton, C (2007)
The Mental Health of Children and Adolescents with Learning Disabilities in Britain. Lancaster: Lancaster University Institute for Health Research.

Fell, F and Hewstone, M (2015)
Psychological Perspectives on Poverty. York: Joseph Rowntree Foundation.

Goddard-Blythe, S (2017)
Attention, Balance and Co-ordination: The ABC of Learning Success. New York, NY: Wiley and Sons.

Goodman, A, Joshi, H, Nasim, B and Tyler, C (2015)
Social and Emotional Skills in Childhood and their Long-Term Effects on Adult Life: A Review for the Early Intervention Foundation. London: Institute of Education/UCL.

Goswami, U (2015)
Children's Cognitive Development and Learning (CPRT Research Survey 3). York: Cambridge Primary Review Trust.

Gray, P (2011)
The Decline of Play and the Rise of Psychopathology in Children and Adolescents. *American Journal of Play,* 3(4).

Grissmer, D, Grimm, K J, Aiyer, S M, Murrah, W M and Steele, J S (2010)
Fine Motor Skills and Early Comprehension of the World: Two New School Readiness Indicators. *Developmental Psychology,* 46(5): 1008–17.

Hackett, L, Theodosiou, L, Bond, C, Blackburn, C and Lever, R (2011)
Understanding the Mental Health Needs of Pupils with Severe Learning Disabilities in an Inner City Local Authority. *British Journal of Learning Disabilities,* 39(4): 327–33.

Hardcastle, K, and Bellis, M (2018)
Routine Enquiry for History of Adverse Childhood Experiences (ACEs) in the Adult Patient Population in a General Practice Setting: A Pathfinder Study. [online] Available at: www.aces.me.uk/ files/2215/3495/0307/REACh_Evaluation_Report.pdf (accessed 9 April 2019).

Hart, S, Logan, J, Soden-Hensler, B, Kershaw, S, Taylor, J and Schatschneider, C (2014)

Exploring How Nature and Nurture Affect the Development of Reading: An Analysis of the Florida Twin Project on Reading. *Development Psychology*, 49(10): 1971–81.

Health and Social Care Information Centre (2018)

Mental Health of Children and Young People in England, 2017 [PAS], NHS Digital. [online] Available at: https://digital.nhs.uk/data-and-information/publications/statistical/mental-health-of-children-and-young-people-in-england/2017/2017 (accessed 28 February 2019).

Heckman, J (2006)

Skill Formation and the Economics of Investing in Disadvantaged Children. Science. *New Series*, 312(5782): 1900–2.

Hill, N and Taylor, L (2004)

Parental School Involvement and Children's Academic Achievement. *American Psychological Society*, 13(4): 161–4.

Hirsh-Pasek, K, Zosh, J, Golinkoff, R M, Gray, J, Robb, M and Kaufman, J (2015)

Putting Education in 'Educational' Apps: Lessons from the Science of Learning. *Psychological Science in the Public Interest*, 16(1): 3–34.

Houghton S, Durkin K, Ang R P, Taylor M F and Brandtman, M (2011)

Measuring Temporal Self-Regulation in Children With and Without Attention Deficit Hyperactivity Disorder – Sense of Time in Everyday Contexts. *European Journal of Psychological Assessment*, 27: 88–94.

House, R (2011)

Too Much Too Soon: Early Learning and the Erosion of Childhood, Stroud: Hawthorn Press.

House of Commons (2018)

The Government's Green Paper on Mental Health: Failing a Generation. London: House of Commons Education and Health and Social Care Committees.

Inness, I (2015)

The Role of Childcare Professionals in Supporting Mental Health and Wellbeing in Young People: A Literature Review. London: Professional Association for Childcare and Early Years.

Jamal, F, Fletcher, A, Harden, A, Wells, H, Thomas, J and Bonell, C (2013)
The School Environment and Student Health: A Systematic Review and Meta-Ethnography of Qualitative Research. *BMC Public Health*, 13(798): 1–11.

James, A, Jenks, C and Prout, A (1998)
Theorizing Childhood. Cambridge: Polity Press.

Jutte, S, Bentley, H, Tallis, D, Mayes, J, Jetha, N, O'Hagan, O, Brookes, H and McConnell, N (2015)
How Safe are Our Children? The Most Comprehensive Overview of Child Protection in the UK. London: NSPCC.

Kangas, J, Ojala, M and Venninen, T (2015)
Children's Self-Regulation in the Context of Participatory Pedagogy in Early Childhood Education. *Early Education and Development*, 26(5–6): 847–70.

The Key (2016)
State of Education Survey. [online] Available at: https://stateofed.thekeysupport.com (accessed 28 February 2019).

Lave, J and Wenger, E (1991)
Situated Learning: Legitimate Peripheral Participation. Cambridge: Cambridge University Press.

Leong, D J and Bodrova, E (2012)
Assessing and Scaffolding Make-Believe Play. *Young Children*, 67(1): 28–34.

Mani, A, Mullainathan, S, Shafir, E and Zhao, J (2013)
Poverty Impedes Cognitive Function. *Science*, 341: 976–80.

Maslow, A H (1943)
A Theory of Human Motivation. *Psychological Review*, 50(4): 370–96.

Maslow, A H (1954)
Motivation and Personality. New York, NY: Harper and Row.

Matthews, T, Danese, A, Wertz, J, Ambler, A, Kelly, M, Diver, A, Caspi, A, Moffitt, T and Arseneault, L (2015)
Social Isolation and Mental Health at Primary and Secondary School Entry: A Longitudinal Cohort Study. *Journal of the American Academy of Child and Adolescent Psychiatry*, 54(3): 225–2.

Mental Health Foundation (MHF) (2016)

Fundamental Facts About Mental Health 2016. [online] Available at: www.mentalhealth.org.uk/sites/default/files/fundamental-facts-about-mental-health-2016.pdf (accessed 9 April 2019).

Minnis, H, Marwick, H, Arthur, J and McLaughlin, A (2006)

Reactive Attachment Disorder: A Theoretical Model Beyond Attachment. *European Child and Adolescent Psychiatry*, 15: 336–42.

Moore, A and Lynch, H (2017)

Understanding a Child's Conceptualisation of Well-Being Through an Exploration of Happiness: The Centrality of Play, People and Place. *Journal of Occupational Science*, 25(1): 124–41.

Moore, T G, Arefadib, N, Deery, A and West, S (2017)

The First Thousand Days: An Evidence Paper. Parkville, Victoria: Centre for Community Child Health, Murdoch Children's Research Institute.

Moyles, J (ed) (2015)

The Excellence of Play (4th edn). Maidenhead: Open University Press.

Murphy, M and Fonagy, P (2013)

Mental Health Problems in Children and Young People. In Davies, S (ed) *Chief Medical Officer Annual Report 2012: Children and Young People's Health: Annual Report on Children and Young People's Health from the Chief Medical Officer (CMO)* (pp 1–13). London: DHSC.

National Collaborating Centre for Mental Health (2015)

Children's Attachment: Attachment in Children and Young People who are Adopted from Care, in Care or at High Risk of Going into Care. [online] Available at: www.nice.org.uk/guidance/NG26/documents/childrens-attachment-full-guideline2 (accessed 9 April 2019).

National Health Service (NHS) (2017)

Mental Health of Children and Young People in England, 2017. [online] Available at: https://digital.nhs.uk/data-and-information/publications/statistical/mental-health-of-children-and-young-people-in-england/2017/2017 (accessed 28 February 2019).

National Institute for Health and Care Excellence (2016)

Children's Attachment. [online] Available at: www.nice.org.uk/guidance/qs133/resources/childrens-attachment-pdf-75545417362885 (accessed 28 February 2019).

Ofsted (2017)

Bold Beginnings: The Reception Curriculum in a Sample of Good and Outstanding Primary Schools. London: Ofsted.

Rasmussen, C (2005)
Executive Functioning and Working Memory in Fetal Alcohol Spectrum Disorder. *Alcoholism: Clinical and Experimental Research*, 29(8): 1359–67.

Roffey, S (2016)
Building a Case for Whole-Child, Whole School Wellbeing in Challenging Contexts. *Educational & Child Psychology*, 33(2): 30–42.

Roffey, S (2017)
'Ordinary Magic' Needs Ordinary Magicians: The Power and Practice of Positive Relationships for Building Youth Resilience and Wellbeing. *Kognition & Pædagogik*, 103.

Rogers, S (ed) (2011)
Rethinking Play and Pedagogy in Early Childhood Education: Concepts, Contexts and Cultures. London: Routledge.

Rüsch, N, Evans-Lacko, S and Thornicroft, D (2012)
What is a Mental Illness? Public Views and Their Effects on Attitudes and Disclosure. *Australian & New Zealand Journal of Psychiatry*, 46(7): 641–50.

Rutter, M (1987)
Psychosocial Resilience and Protective Mechanisms. *American Journal of Orthopsychiatry*, 57(3): 316–31.

Saeri, A, Cruwys, T, Barlow, F, Stronge, S and Sibley, C (2017)
Social Connectedness Improves Public Mental Health: Investigating Bidirectional Relationships in the New Zealand Attitudes and Values Survey. *Australian & New Zealand Journal of Psychiatry*, 52(4): 365–74.

Schumacher, J, Hoffman, P, Schmal, C, Schulte-Korne, G and Nothen, M (2007)
Genetics of Dyslexia: The Evolving Landscape. *Journal of Medical Genetics*, 44(5): 289–97.

Snowling, M J, Hulme, C, Bailey A M, Stothard, S E and Lindsay, G (2011)
Better Communication Research Programme: Language and Literacy Attainment of Pupils During Early Years and Through KS2: Does Teacher Assessment at Five Provide a Valid Measure of Children's Current and Future Educational Attainments? DfE Research Brief DFE-RB 172a. London: DfE Publications.

Stewart, N and Pugh, R (2007)
Early Years Vision in Focus, Part 3: Exploring Pedagogy. Shrewsbury: Shropshire County Council.

Stratton, K, Howe, C and Battaglia, F (1996)
Fetal Alcohol Syndrome: Epidemiology, Prevention, and Treatment.
Washington, DC: National Academy Press.

Sylva, K, Melhuish, E, Sammons, P, Siraj-Blatchford, I and Taggart, B (2004)
The Effective Provision of Pre-School Education Project: Findings from Pre-School to End of Key Stage 1. London: Institute of Education.

Taggart, L, Cousins, W and Milner, S (2007)
Young People with Learning Disabilities Living in State Care: Their Emotional, Behavioural and Mental Health Status. *Child Care in Practice*, 13(4): 401–16.

Taket, A, Stagnitti, K, Nolan, A and Casey, S (2012)
Preschool Teachers' Strategies for Supporting Resilience in Early Childhood. *Professional Voice*, 9(1): 39–45.

Tickell, C (2011)
The Early Years: Foundations for Life, Health and Learning. London: Crown Copyright. [online] Available at: www.gov.uk/government/publications/the-early-years-foundations-for-life-health-and-learning-an-independent-report-on-the-early-years-foundation-stage-to-her-majestys-government (accessed 28 February 2019).

Tovey, H (2010)
Playing on the Edge: Perceptions of Risk and Danger in Outdoor Play. In Broadhead, P, Howard, J and Wood, E (eds), *Play and Learning in the Early Years* (pp 79–94). London: Sage.

Vygotsky, L S (1967)
Play and Its Role in the Mental Development of the Child. *Soviet Psychology*, 5: 6–18.

Vygotsky, L S (1978)
Mind in Society: The Development of Higher Psychological Processes. Cambridge, MA: Harvard University Press.

Whitebread, D and Bingham, S (2014)
School Readiness: Starting Age, Cohorts and Transitions in the Early Years. In Moyles, J, Georgeson, J and Payler, J (eds) *Early Years Foundations: Critical Issues* (2nd edn) (pp 179–91). Maidenhead: Open University Press.

Whitebread, D (2012)
The Importance of Play. [online] Available at: www.importanceofplay.eu/IMG/pdf/dr_david_whitebread_-_the_importance_of_play.pdf (accessed 28 February 2019).

Wood, D, Bruner, J and Ross, G (1976)
The Role of Tutoring in Problem Solving. *Journal of Child Psychology and Child Psychiatry*, 17: 89–100.

Zosh, J M, Hopkins, E J, Jensen, H, Liu, C, Neale, D, Hirsh-Pasek, K, Solis, S L, and Whitebread, D (2017)
Learning Through Play: A Review of the Evidence (White Paper). London: The LEGO Foundation/DK.

+INDEX